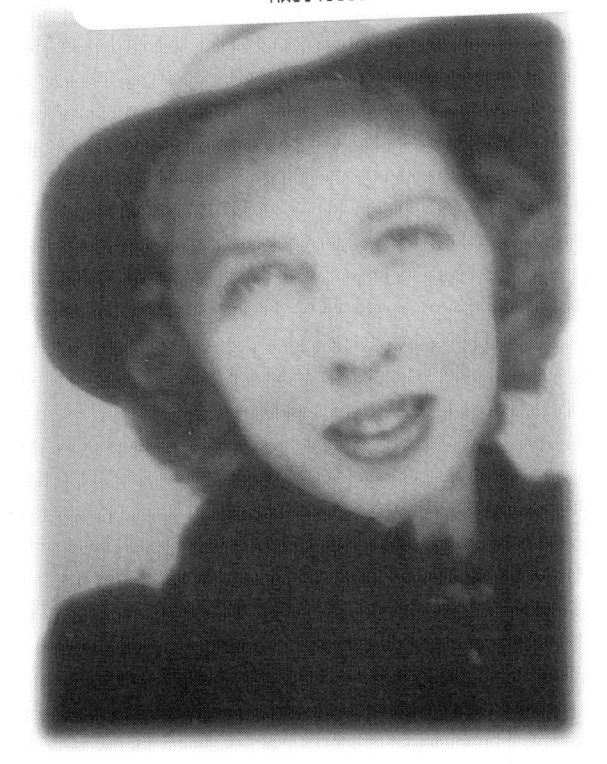

Excerpts from

Elsie at Ebb Tide:
Emerging from the Undertow of Alzheimer's

Barbara Erakko

*Dedicated to my mother
who went so unwillingly
into Alzheimer's
yet taught me so much about love
and the eternal dance between body and spirit*

*And to every soul
who enters into this strange portal
that pushes past mind
and memory*

© All Rights Reserved 2015
Bella Barbara Erakko
ISBN 13: 978-1515334132

Preface

Alzheimer's is a terrifying disease. When my mother began her 13-year journey through Alzheimer's, both of us expected a fearful descent into mindlessness. We made the best of it. Mom fought with all her intelligence; I struggled to keep her safe, healthy, and more importantly, *alive*

For many years, that worked. But it also blinded us to another story unfolding right beneath our eyes—within our hearts. It took a crisis to open a very unexpected door.

One day, my mother's face looked contorted with agony. Was she in pain? Should I call 911? I no longer had any way to communicate. Desperate, I realized I knew one person, a friend, who might help—a medical intuitive who used psychic abilities to identify illness.

Truly it was a leap in the dark. Who, after all, had tried telepathic communication in cases of advanced Alzheimer's? I certainly knew of no one! But it is no cliché to say that desperate times call for desperate measures. I was desperate.

I took the leap. I asked my friend to telepathically connect with my mother.

Mom did not need 911 in a medical sense that day. She needed 911 in an emotional sense—and my friend Kenna, to my surprise, became her paramedic, in a paranormal way. She developed a relationship with Mom, who shared insights and bits of her life telepathically.

In 2014, I published *Elsie at Ebb Tide: Emerging from the Undertow of Alzheimer's*. This 465-page book intertwines three stories: My mother's life as a Finnish American woman who became a U.S. Protocol Officer for the State Department; her journey through Alzheimer's; and lastly, what unfolded when Kenna, Mom, and I explored telepathic communication.

I kept verbatim transcripts of every session between Kenna and my mother, who died in 2000. They are included here.

Feeling I was already "out on a limb," I took one step further. I decided to ask five experienced psychics to interview Mom on the other side, to seek answers to two questions:

1) What was her experience of Alzheimer's from the inside out?
2) What would she want caregivers to know?

Mom answered the questions in very consistent ways. She also offered, of her own accord, how it felt to die. And she always included particular "identifiers" so I would know it was Elsie. All of that information is included here.

Alzheimer's: Living Between Body and Spirit focuses solely on the telepathic aspects of my mother's experience of Alzheimer's. It delves into the question of whether soul-to-soul communication is possible when the brain no longer functions.

It asks, and suggests the answer to the question, *Can spirit emerge from the rubble of a ruined mind?*

Introduction

Elsie Nurmi died on Friday, October 13, 2000—enough into the new millennium to firmly plant her feet and say, "I made it," but not long enough to make much of a dent. She became a very reluctant member of a long family line stricken with Alzheimer's.

I feel, in some ways, those last years were the best for both of us. We had more fun; we laughed more. She resisted the disease with aplomb, insisting she never be told she had it. As her memory faded, she knew enough to ask me to get her a new brain. "Can't you find a doctor for that, Barbara?"

She also knew enough to hurtle cold fury at me when I attempted to manage her care in ways she didn't like, icily telling me, "I *never* used the word 'love' with you. I don't really like you."

I watched her life peel away, like an onion. First to go were the names of friends and her how-to-do-it knowledge. Sandra and I, her two daughters, dropped off the memory tree soon after like overripe fruit.

The memory of Herby, her deceased husband, languished for a while. Then it, too, was gone. Last to go and most slowly was the memory of her job and her name

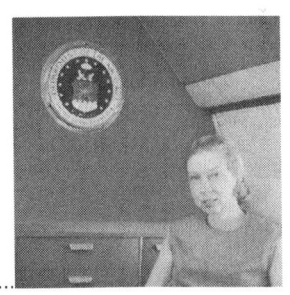

Elsie Julia Elizabeth Norlund Nurmi,
Protocol Officer, U.S. Department of State

She led American delegations overseas using presidential aircraft. She attended coronations, private audiences with the pope, and met queens. When heads of state visited the United States, she coordinated hotels, food, and travel. In such heady circumstances, what surprised her most were the funny human moments such as mistaking Nixon for hotel staff.

But then her memory slipped. Was she *in* the motorcade when Kennedy died? In the car behind him? Or (in reality) *at her desk in the State Department*? ... She told everyone who saw the personally signed presidential photos that she was part of history. Yet she couldn't quite remember which part. But eventually it no longer mattered. She forgot it all.

As she forgot *this* world, she began to see into another world. She caught up with old friends visiting from the other side. Strangely, only the deceased paid social calls in this between-land. She'd point them out, frustrated that we couldn't see them.

These forays seemed nice, like postcards from the future, a future we all will encounter one day.

As the thirteen-year-long disease progressed, I began to observe something remarkable happening. Mom became more honest. No longer able to be polite, her yeses and noes came from all that was left of her—an unvarnished, unadorned soul.

As I sat by her side talking to her as though she were entirely aware, I felt she *was* entirely there—and aware. I conversed with her *spirit*, knowing that it was immutable and simply trapped in a diseased body. Eventually, in the last year of her life when anyone might believe nothing of Elsie remained, I believed *all* of Elsie remained.

As the disease ravaged her body, I saw and felt a pure soul emerging. Quite remarkable, it seemed as shocking in some respects as a caterpillar melting down to liquid in a cocoon only to emerge as a butterfly.

The last time I saw her, she grasped my forearms and gazed directly into my eyes with startling clarity, the fog gone. Suddenly I saw something I had never seen—not in her eyes or any eyes. It was as though pure consciousness poured through her. I saw what she now saw. I was looking right into Spirit—pure Love unfettered by a human body. She allowed me to see the whole cosmos of Love pouring through her. I was literally knocked out of my senses. Rather than "lights out," I witnessed *transcendent lights on.*

It shook me to my core and left me in unquenchable awe. I realized something quite remarkable lay buried beneath the rubble of this disease. One could almost *see* body turn into spirit.

I knew, as did my sister Sandra, that when she decided to go, it would be fast. On October 13, 2000, the call came. Mom was dying.

In hours, poof! She was gone. Passport expired.

Elsie (1917-2000)

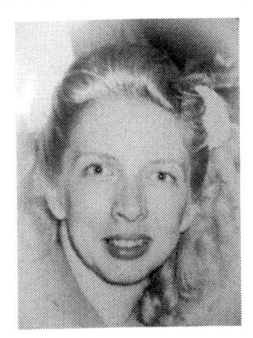

Elsie

The heroine of her own life, Elsie writes letters to herself as a child and stuffs them into the barn wall until one year the mice eat them. Speaking only Finnish, she rides in a horse-drawn prairie wagon to a two-room school in Finlayson, Minnesota, but ends up flying on presidential aircraft.

She leaves Minnesota at the age of 19, ending her nanny job and her attendance at the Duluth Business School. Offered a free ride to New York City, she becomes a live-in "butler's girl" for a Wall Street executive's family. Using her meager earnings, she continues business school, garnering shorthand skills and launching herself through seven clerical jobs in rapid succession.

Meanwhile, she dances the schottische at the Harlem Finnish Dance Hall and meets Herby—the man who turns every Finnish girl's eye.

When he disappears mysteriously from her life, she takes federal employment with the Census Bureau in Washington, D.C. Months later, after grieving and burying his mother, Herby shows up unexpectedly on her doorstep. Marriage soon follows and she continues in the workplace until their first child, Sandra, is born, and two years later, Barbara.

Rejoining the federal work force with the excuse she needs Christmas money, Elsie works for the Panama Canal offices in D.C., then the State Department.

There, she inventories gifts given to U.S. citizens by foreign governments, eventually moving to the Office of Protocol. There, she manages foreign state visits to the United States and presidential delegations abroad, flying to every continent except Antarctica.

Accompanying the official delegations, she meets queens, kings, popes, heads of state, and even a would-be assassin. She oversees dinners, rides in ticker tape parades, and maintains a "security system" allowing access to White House grounds—a custom-designed enamel lapel pin.

And sometimes, things don't go as planned.

When a head of state and his wife arrive by helicopter for a White House arrival ceremony, Elsie stands patiently beside Lady Bird Johnson holding a bouquet of long-stemmed red roses. The copter blades create a deafening roar, but once on the ground quietly rotate.

Elsie looks down to give the flowers one last check. To her horror, hundreds of red rose petals are fluttering across the lawn, leaving Elsie with a bouquet of flowerless stems, and an empty-handed First Lady.

Then there is the assassination attempt. President Tito of Yugoslavia faces a threat on his life in a five-star New York City hotel on a visit where Elsie is the Protocol Officer in charge. She attends the smoke-filled interrogation of the captured assailant and reluctantly reads a press release, in her bathrobe, as Tito is rapidly and unceremoniously returned to his country.

At any rate, after twenty-five years, she retires with Herby to Florida. Eventually widowed and after a lifetime of travel, she faces a journey she never expected—one into mindlessness. It becomes her most transcendent destination.

She holds onto life until Friday, October 13, 2000, then lets go of it in a lightning flash.

Barbara

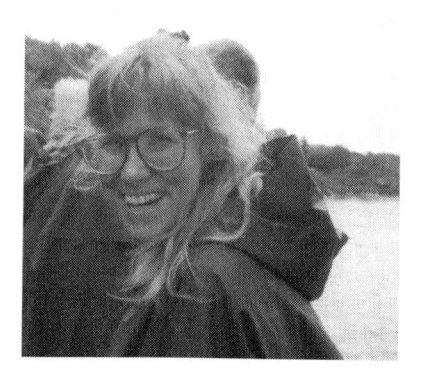

The younger of two daughters, Barbara becomes Elsie's care manager while Sandra, who lives 3,000 miles away, supports Barbara emotionally.

Some of the roughest transitions occur during the early years of the disease.

Elsie refuses to admit she has Alzheimer's, though it runs through her Norlund family. When Barbara suggests testing, explaining that the memory loss could be due to mini-strokes or nutritional issues, Elsie reluctantly agrees.

But when the diagnosis comes back, she lashes out at her daughter, refusing for a time to even see her.

The necessary move from Florida to Maryland also infuriates Elsie, who icily tells Barbara, "You go your way; I'll go mine," before slamming her door shut in Barbara's face.

Once in Maryland, in various care facilities over the next several years, the mother-daughter relationship moves into smoother waters.

As Elsie slowly stops fighting the disease, her playfulness, wit, and wisdom peek out. Barbara sees a mother she never knew—the woman who her father Herby had fallen so deeply in love with, long ago.

Eventually, when Elsie falls, breaking her hip due to advanced osteoporosis, Barbara brings her into her own home for care. The doctors predict Elsie will not live one year. Hiring a caregiver to help with day-to-day tasks, Barbara expects the worst ... a bedridden incoherent woman in the final stages of a devastating disease.

But something quite different happens...

The Story Begins...

To understand this very unusual story which follows, one must go back in time.

Barbara and her older sister Sandra grew up in a family where logic and science predominated. It wouldn't be an understatement to say that Einstein held far more sway than poetry or art in their father Herby's eyes. Every member of the family developed superior left brain analytical talents.

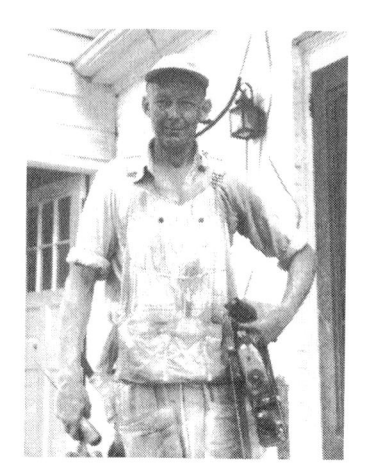

Herby (1913-1987)

Herby, a self-employed carpenter with a probable genius IQ, read and reread Einstein's Theory of Relativity. He doggedly tried to master it in his lifetime, albeit without a background in physics. Elsie used her extraordinary organizational ability to manage delegations visiting U.S. presidents and lead White House delegations abroad. Sandra graduated from college with a language degree, got a second degree in electrical engineering, and took a civilian job with the U.S. Navy. Barbara acquired a master's degree in library science, and designed information systems.

The intuitive, artistic, sensitive right brain received little if any attention from the Nurmi family. But all of that would change for Barbara, and eventually, for Elsie...

Trying Something New in Key West

I gaze out the car window with the ecstasy only a frozen snowbird can feel as I head out of Miami. I'm on my way to visit my friend Rosemary in Key West.

I even enjoy the rotten-fish smell that sometimes floats through my open window.

As I drive, I think about Rosemary's unusual life. Once married to a disc jockey who became a medical-magazine salesman and eventually launched his own magazine, Rosemary went from frugal housewife and salaried nurse to a woman in fur and pearls.

But now, decades later, her husband deceased, her children grown, she lives in an eclectic cottage with her own art studio filled with large colorful canvases.

What alternative healing thing is she into now? I wonder. With that thought, I make a rash decision. *Whatever she is into, I'll try it.* I know it'll be different, interesting, perhaps even weird.

Rosemary, her face framed in wavy dark hair with silver streaks, opens the door, her smile lighting up her dark brown eyes. I walk into her magical world.

Right in front of me, on the wall, a huge vibrant-colored horse cut out of paper fills an area over six feet in length. Everywhere I turn, I see the color and light of an artist radiating out of this home. Each dining-room chair has its own painted design; the tiled table pops with energy.

That evening, as we sit in her living room under magnificent pieces of collage and abstract art, I ask, "So what type of healing are you doing these days?"

"Ohhhh, Barbara," she exclaims. "I've been working with an energy healer. She's *wonderful.*"

"Yeah, but what is energy healing?"

She walks over to her birch wood bookcase and pulls off *Hands of Light* by Barbara Brennan, handing me the book as she tries to explain.

"She grew up on a Wisconsin farm and often went into the woods by herself. She would sit very still—even animals would approach her. Over time she learned she could sense things—like closing her eyes and knowing where a tree would be before she could touch it. The more she did it, the better she got.

"It was like she was feeling the *energy* of the trees and the animals."

Rosemary took the book and opened it to a well-marked page. "She was sensing their energy auras, and she used the example of candle light to explain it. Here it is: 'Consider the candle and its flame. ... Where does the light begin and where does the flame end? There seems to be a line here but where exactly is it?'"

Listening to Brennan's words, I try to wrap my brain around this analogy.

"Oh," I look up. "When I'm thinking a thought—like I've got to go to the grocery store—I'm the flame. It's a concrete thought and kind of like a flame. You can see the beginning and end of it. It has edges. But if, for example, I'm looking at a sunset and I sort of lose myself in the moment, then I don't know where 'I' begin and this sense of awe—this expanded state—begins."

"It's like she's asking us to think a different way," Rosemary suggests, "but it's not like she understood what was happening to her as a child.

"She got older, stopped going into the woods, and kind of forgot about it." Rosemary laughed. "She got a master's degree in atmospheric physics and worked for NASA.

"Eventually she became a counselor. She started seeing energies around her clients, but by now her scientific training made her skeptical so she just kept observing.

She says: 'I saw that the energy field is intimately associated with a person's health and well-being. If a person is unhealthy, it will show in his energy field as an unbalanced flow of energy and/or stagnated energy.'"

Rosemary closed the book and handed it back to me. "Anyway, she found herself receiving channeled information. For example, she began to see cancer in people very clearly—and subsequent medical tests proved her right.

"She could also assist the healing process by rebalancing the client's field. She said that many times illness has a psychological or physical trauma associated with it, and in order to completely heal, the person must also address that issue."

"Well, do you work with her?" I ask.

"No, but one of her students who trained for four years under her works in Key West. She comes to my house and I get healings about once a month."

There! I think to myself. I picked something new.

Two days later, a soft-spoken Emily shows up with her massage table. I lay down and she begins, scarcely touching me.

I feel gentle fingers on my feet, sometimes a light touch on my body. I slip into a deep peacefulness no longer caring what she does.

When at last I slowly sit up she tells me, "Your body is very divided, as though your waist was cut right through the middle, as though you haven't totally agreed to be on earth. I suspect you have trouble grounding yourself."

When someone says something to you that you've never heard in your life, either it resonates with your inner knowing or it doesn't. *You are so right,* I immediately know.

An image flashes through my mind and I share it. "This goes back to my birth. I am sure of it. It's as though I got born and all of the sudden realized I had made a *huge* mistake.

I was like this little baby with my feet crabbed up against my butt screaming *BEAM ME BACK UP! I MADE A MISTAKE!* And then I realized I was stuck here. But I never put my feet down."

"Well, Barbara," Emily suggests, "you might want to try. After all it is amazing to have a human body. We have hands and feet and a mind; we can do so much on earth."

When I share the experience with Rosemary, I decide that when I get back to Maryland, I will find another Brennan graduate and try this again. It is a decision that will change my life, even my way of looking at it. More surprising, it will change the way I look at Alzheimer's.

A Different Way of Healing

Not forgetting my promise, I decide to interview three Barbara Brennan graduates.

My first telephone call is to a woman named Kenna. "Hello," I begin, "I understand you are a Barbara Brennan graduate."

"Yes, I am," Kenna replies in a voice that sounds like a little wren.

"Do you have an office?"

"No."

"How do you work, then?"

"Oh, I come to your home."

"Do you have a massage table that you use?"

"Oh no, I'm too *little*. I couldn't carry it. You see, I'm not even five feet tall."

"So how do you work?"

"Oh, you lie on your dining-room table."

"Let me think about it. I'm interviewing two other Brennan graduates."

"Well, if you're meant to work with me, it'll just happen," Kenna cheerily answers, ending the conversation. No sales pitch. No "Let's set an appointment." No discounted six-treatment plan.

I find Kenna intriguing and the others much less so. They *do* have offices. They offer different modalities of healing, everything from massage to psychotherapy to Reiki. Brennan's approach simply is another tool in their healing kits. Kenna banks her life on it.

I choose Kenna.

~ ~ ~

The day for the healing arrives. I hear a knock on my door and throw it open.

Gazing down at Kenna, I say, "My *god*, you *are* small!"

She stands before me, blue eyes twinkling, a tiny gnome of a person dressed all in mauve, her light brown hair softly curled into a pageboy that perfectly frames her heart-shaped face. Soon we are ready.

"Just lay quietly," Kenna tells me. As Kenna begins her work, I close my eyes but peek out of them once in a while.

She scarcely touches me. She stands at my feet gently placing her hands on their tops. I feel ripples running down my body toward her. Suddenly I *relax*. The scared tension I've been holding drains out of me like water from a tub.

After awhile, she moves to my right side. I see her waving her arms over me.

If I were sitting on the sofa watching, I'd think she was a Druid priestess performing some bizarre rite. But this is *me* she is working on!

Again I feel a strange but pleasant rippling over my belly and chest. I fall asleep and remember nothing else. I have no idea how much time has passed, but suddenly and very gently I awake.

Kenna is now behind me. I feel tingling in my head though she is not touching me. Then it is over. I see Kenna sitting on a dining-room chair near me writing in her notebook. I lay in bliss. I feel as though I've experienced a deep *inside* massage, everything calm within me.

I eventually learn that some people experience more, some less. Those who are naturally psychic may even see the auras themselves. They *feel* the healing more directly.

My experience never goes beyond this sense of ripples and tingling, of being drawn deeply into my body, and experiencing an overwhelming sense of Love pouring in as though I am being *filled* with Light.

Later Kenna tells me the same thing Emily had—"Barbara, you are *very* ungrounded. It took me almost 20 minutes to get you into your body."

I sense the difference. Rather than breathing in a shallow slightly anxious way, I now draw deep breaths. I feel safe, grounded, peaceful—unusual sensations for me.

For people naturally grounded, it must be almost impossible to understand how ungroundedness feels. But for those of us whose defense mechanism is flight rather than fight, energetically speaking we truly *know* the difference, and it feels *good* to be home in our bodies.

How Far Can Energy Healing Travel?

"Let's go on another trip," I suggest to my older friend Anita.

After much discussion, we agree on Chicago and Niagara Falls but by the second day my right shoulder hurts so badly I can scarcely drive. Unable to sleep, I am getting more and more tired. We still have ten days of vacation to go.

Considering my options, I recall a recent conversation with Kenna where she talked about experimenting with long-distance healing.

What have I got to lose, I decide, *except a little money if it doesn't work?*

We agree to work the next day at 5 a.m. central time when hopefully I'll be asleep. I'm not. I struggle to relax, then suddenly—just as though she were actually there—I feel the familiar rippling, the deep relaxation. I fall asleep.

When I wake two hours later, I slowly sit up and rotate my arm. It's tender, but the sharp pain is completely gone. *Maybe just coincidence,* I admit, *but it's a huge difference.*

"Kenna," I call to thank her, "I think I'm okay." Once again, I want to know how she does this, especially long distance. "I just don't get it," I tell her.

"Oh," she laughs, "I don't know how to explain it. How is it that we are talking right now? We could talk about how the brain sends the signal to the mouth and tongue and how vibrations or waves go from your mouth into my ear."

I laugh. "I give up. Put that way, talking sounds just as strange."

Over time, Kenna and I will work exclusively this way. She saves travel time; I relax more deeply in my own bed.

I still feel the rippling waves, the tingling, the experience of Light flowing in. I have the same grounded sensation and sense of deep interior massage. *I don't have to understand how this works,* I occasionally tell myself.

Despite my scientific analytical nature that wants to intellectually understand, I realize my body responds to energy healing without any left-brain support from me.

Eventually, a crisis will catapult me and my mother into a much deeper experience of long-distance healing, and telepathic communication. But that moment is six years away...

Letting Go

Meanwhile, month by month, year by year, Mom loses ground to the disease until, in the eleventh year she falls and breaks her hip. The doctor tells me she very likely will die within the year.

Looking at her sleeping in a darkened rehab room, with cold oatmeal congealing by her side and her head hanging unnaturally off the bed, I realize that without my help, she will die in far less than a year.

I stand in her darkened room, silently asking her ... *is it your time?*

I decide *no*, and hire a live-in caregiver, Hawa, a native of Sierra Leone, to help me.

I am bringing Mom home.

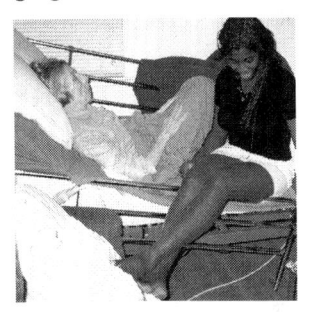

When Mom first came into my house, if anything bad happened to her, I would have taken her to the hospital in a New York minute. I would have called 911 and had her whisked away—and cured.

Then I slowly realized her body had passed a portal. I posted a DO NOT RESUSCITATE order on the front door. Every bone in her rib cage would break with the slightest pressure. My new mantra became *over my dead body will she experience pain*. I began to let her lead; I learned to follow....

I let go of the retirement home in Florida.

I let go of the Alzheimer's facility in Maryland.

I let go of the group home.

I let go of resuscitation.

As she let go, I learned to let go.

I've let go of her laughter, her naughty playful eyes.

I've let go of her wakefulness.

I've let go of her coherence, and her saying I am beautiful.

Wherever she goes, I follow, fascinated.

When she goes into deep sleep, a slumber beyond slumber, I stand at her bedside wondering, *where are you now?*

To my surprise, she continues to lead, as always a mother.

And I, as always a daughter, follow.

But now, something is about to change for both of us.

I poke my head into her bedroom. Finding her awake, I bend over to look into her eyes. She gazes back at me like a trapped terrified animal.

"Mom, what's *wrong*?" I ask the one question she cannot answer.

I begin to panic. *Is she in pain? What if she needs to go to the emergency room?*

I feel completely helpless. I will my mind to find a way into hers.

18

I keep staring at her, increasingly anxious ... and in that moment the thought of *Kenna* flies into my mind.

"Mom," I say, "I'll be right back. I need to make a call." I rush from the room. As I hurry to the phone, I tell myself, *Kenna can connect with Mom.*

I make the call that will change everything about the way I think about Alzheimer's.

~ ~ ~

"Kenna," a whirlwind of words pours out my mouth, "Mom's in trouble. Something's wrong and I don't know what. She may be in physical pain, or she's in some awful nightmare. Can you connect with her right away and find out what's happening."

"I'll have to ask her permission, Barbara."

"I know," I answer.

Kenna's standards for intervention are high. She treats each soul with the greatest respect. Mom, though damaged by Alzheimer's, still retains an intact functioning spirit. Kenna will be connecting with that higher self, asking permission to visit.

Now I have to wait. I pace. I wash dishes. I try to sit and calm myself. At last the phone rings.

"Your mother was very anxious, Barbara. When I asked her why, she said, 'I don't know where I am. I'm afraid I'm dying.' I explained everything to her. I think you'll find she's calmer now."

Overwhelmed with relief, I hang up. When I return, I find Mom's face once again calm, her eyes quiet and seemingly lost; she has returned to the only normalcy I know—Alzheimer's.

After this frightening episode, my sister Sandra and I agree. We hire Kenna to connect regularly with Mom.

We reserve judgment. It may be "real"; it may be sheer fantasy. But if it gives Mom comfort, we are willing to explore this avenue of communication. "I'll write down whatever Kenna tells me," I promise my sister.

And so, a door opens.

Is It Today or Tomorrow?

As I set the appointment between Elsie and Kenna, I turn over questions in my mind. *Will we know if it's really Elsie? What do I want to ask her? Does this help her?* I see it as an experiment. I have few if any expectations other than a *hope* that Kenna can indeed meet with Mom on a spirit level.

When Kenna asks me, "Do you have anything you want to know from your mother?" At first I say no but then I pause, "Kenna, we have no idea what she wants for a funeral. Does she want to be cremated or buried? Does she have any special songs she wants at her memorial service? We never asked her and now it seems too late."

"Well," Kenna offers, "Let's see what she says."

~ ~ ~

Elsie: I want to kick up my heels and ride out of here. I just want to move. I feel like fish soup. Once the fish is in the soup, it's not likely to go anywhere else.

Kenna: You can go places in your mind.

Elsie: Yes, that's the only book I read now. Reading the mind with its jumbled pages. Short stories instead of a long novel.

Kenna: I'm experiencing these little scenes with you, Elsie.

Elsie: *I feel lost and found. You can always find me here in this body but my mind is often lost.*

Elsie: *Why doesn't Sandra come to visit?*

Kenna: She is far away.

Elsie: *I'm getting old and I am not really enjoying this. I am all right but this is no fun. Sometimes I feel like I will be here forever whether I want to be or not.*

Kenna: Yes, but you are staying.

Elsie: *I feel safe here.*

Kenna: I can help you feel safe on the other side.

Elsie: *I am not ready yet.*

Elsie: *My thoughts used to be quite orderly. I liked plans, knowing what to expect when. Now time runs together for me, like rivers into oceans. Is it today or yesterday? Time is something I have so much of, but I do not know what to do with it or where to put it. I do not need to save it because it is always available. The monotony is unbelievable and I am a part of it. I used to be very busy, but now is now.*

Kenna: Do you want to tell Barbara anything?

Elsie: *I'm actually okay. I'm feeling better. I want to tell her that it is not just that I do not make any sense but not much of anything makes sense, so how can I?*

Kenna: Do you want me to help you here, or there?

Elsie: *I don't know. I like the in-between.*

Kenna: Barbara worries about what you will want for your funeral.

Elsie: You know it really does not matter that much to me now. I suppose a church is nicer and Barbara would like it, don't you think? But I am really only interested in music. I still want to dance, you know. I like piano better than organ.

Elsie: You can bury ashes, can't you? I certainly could stand being a little warmer. Then, I don't know. Whatever is easier for Barbara. I used to worry about such details.

Kenna: You have lots of family [deceased] around you. You can tell the angels what you need and they will help you.

Elsie: My husband liked the beach. My days are like this. Reminiscing.

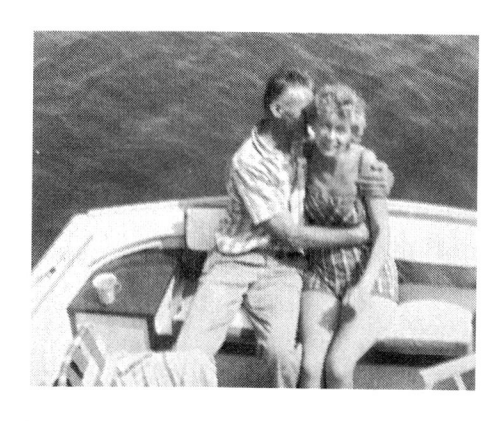

Kenna: Is there anything I can do for you?

Elsie: Can you sing?

Kenna: I really cannot sing. But I will sing a little lullaby.

Kenna: There are four angels. Can you see them?

Elsie: No, but I feel them.

~ ~ ~

As I listen to Kenna read her notes about her conversation with Elsie, I am struck by how a new relationship begins.

Mom speaks in her trademark somewhat-humorous voice. She's an action person. *I want to kick up my heels.*

Kenna prefers the subtle spiritual approach ... *You can go places in your mind.*

Clearly, Elsie doesn't know much about that world. She begins by talking about fish soup, something Americans would rarely if ever eat but something with which Finns would be well acquainted.

She explains to Kenna that Herby loved the beach. True. She tells Kenna she loves to dance. True. That she prefers the piano to the organ. True. She always owned a piano and played it, while she only used the organ during her teen years for the Finlayson church.

When asked about funeral arrangements, she admits she no longer cares much about it. The woman who designed her own monument down to its last chiseled letter admits *I used to worry about such details.*

To my surprise, she asks about burying ashes.

Sandra and I have presumed, having no guidance from her, that she preferred burial because she wanted to wear the black suit she wore when meeting Pope Paul VI.

But now she jokes, *I certainly could stand being a little warmer.* "So what do we do?" I later ask my sister.

"I think she wants to be with Dad in every way," Sandra answers. "He was cremated. It makes her feel closer to him."

Knowing our mother, that makes absolute sense. She will be buried in accordance with her long-standing wishes in Finlayson Lutheran Cemetery. But not in body—in ashes.

Most important from a caregiving perspective, I learn her level of awareness. I find myself reassured by Mom's words, *I am not ready*, when Kenna says she can help her to feel safe on the other side. I feel I made the right decision bringing her home.

When I stood in that darkened rehab room silently wondering if Mom was ready to let go, I felt her spirit too strong, too vibrant. It just wasn't time. Now, she even wonders why Sandra is not visiting.

I feel for the first time that we have a link to Elsie—a way, however tenuous, to communicate. A process begins that we will use until Mom dies. In fact, Kenna will be connected to my mother within an hour of her death, and then within hours, on the other side.

The Cluttered Room

Kenna continues to give me clues about how she receives information. One day she tells me, "Oh, it's like Dr. Spock."

Thinking of the show *Star Trek,* I ask, "You mean when he touches another person's head and the two minds temporarily meld?"

"Yes. It's as though I see what your mother sees." And so, the second conversation with Elsie begins...

~ ~ ~

Elsie: *Know what I've been thinking about? About all the time I have now. And when I could make use of it, I didn't have it. Now I can't do much with it. I do get bored but what can I do? The pleasures and pains of old age—I have to accept it. There's nothing else to do.*

Kenna: What's in your heart tonight?

Elsie: Oh, I like the piano. I wish I could play it and dance like I used to. Dancing is not just exercise for the body; it's a way to clear the mind too.

Kenna: You seem tired.

Elsie: I got a chill a few days ago.

[Kenna did brain balancing. She could see that her brain looked like dead-end streets—no information could go through.]

Elsie: [referring to her brain, said]: You could make a playroom out of it.

Kenna: What do you mean?

Elsie: You know how a child plays with a toy and then leaves it and goes to the next and leaves it and the room can get cluttered with toys—but there's no one to clean up my play room. The toys are left there to clutter my mind. I can't walk through easily.

I can't find what I'm looking for. I generally have to wait until I bump into it. It becomes like a new discovery. I know there's so much in my mind, but I can't find it when I want to.

Kenna: We can clean out the clutter.

Elsie: Thank you. Thank Barbara too. When is she coming back? I've forgotten.

Kenna: In a few days.

~ ~ ~

As I write down Kenna's conversation with Mom in the hotel room, I keep one anxious eye on the clock.

I'm running late for a meeting but I want to hear everything. As soon as we hang up, I grab my purse and keys and dash out the door.

Once I ease into traffic, I mull over Mom's comments: *"I like the piano. I wish I could play it and dance like I used to."*

Tears sting my eyes. Mom loved music. Her simple way of speaking, so familiar to me, matches the way she responded to life.

But I also notice how Kenna, as Elsie's translator, sometimes uses her own vocabulary for describing things.

Mom never said she "had a chill" (she always had a "cold").

As I think back to Kenna's Dr. Spock image, I realize that somehow Elsie telepathically conveys her thoughts to Kenna. Kenna may see Mom dancing and pointing to her body and then her mind and then Kenna hears phrases like *exercise* and *clear mind*.

It's up to Kenna to match what she's receiving with a specific translation I might understand. Mom lives in a different world now, one dependent on oblique communication.

I continue to think about dancing.

Maybe that was the only way she could let go and just enjoy herself without worry, without being responsible all the time, I tell myself.

I am struck by Mom's image of a cluttered toy room. It seems some aspect of Elsie (her soul? her spirit?) remains undiseased. She can describe how she uses her wits in an increasingly witless situation: *"I can't find what I'm looking for. I generally have to wait until I bump into it."*

Later, I will read about how neuroscientist Dr. Jill Taylor, who suffers a devastating stroke, recovers and gives a very similar explanation. But now, in many respects, Kenna is Mom's only portal to the outside world.

I Want to Dance

Kenna and Mom are slowly establishing a relationship. In a way, the conversations become more concrete—about everyday things, wishes and needs.

~ ~ ~

Elsie: *I don't feel like I will be living much longer. I am feeling weak.*

Kenna: Why?

Elsie: *I don't know. I am just weaker than before. I feel strange.*

Kenna: You could live much longer.

Elsie: I'm just growing more tired of being here like this.

Kenna: What would you like?

Elsie: *I want to leave something for my grandchildren. I want them to remember me.*

Kenna: I'll tell Barbara.

Elsie: Well, Barbara can do anything. Don't tell her she can't—that is just when she will! Can you tell Barbara to hold my hands more? It is only when I am touched that I know that I am here.

[Kenna starts to cry as she begins to fill Elsie with Light.]

Elsie: Oh, that feels so good.

Kenna: So what's in your heart, Elsie?

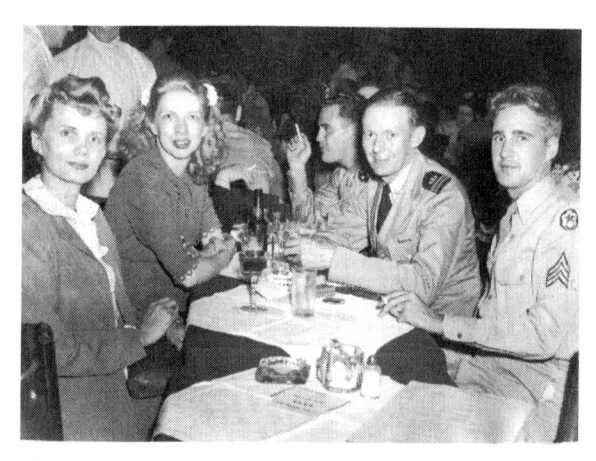

Elsie: I want to dance. I wish I could. I liked to fly. But my husband preferred the water and boats. Sandra and Barbara have been good daughters. I am like an old leaf on a tree.

Kenna: Can you see angels, Elsie?

Elsie: Yes. I am seeing them now. I am getting tired. I will be ready when Barbara is ready.

Kenna: Would you like me to come back to visit?

Elsie: The door is always open. Right now I want to get some sleep.

~ ~ ~

After Kenna finishes her session with Mom, we talk and I write down the messages.

I go into Mom's room and watch her as she sleeps with her face at peace, her mouth ever so slightly open, a tiny smile seeming to tug at the corners.

Perhaps you are talking with the angels, I think. *Or maybe you're flying on Air Force Two*. Kenna received one message clearly: Dad loved water; Mom loved air. How true.

I wonder about her words, *I will be ready when Barbara is ready.*

Does she know how I've fretted about the funeral? Strangely, even during these declining stages, I still find moments when she seems briefly lucid.

About 2 weeks ago, I walked in and saw her cheeks wet with tears. I bent over her and asked, "What's wrong, Mom?" To my surprise she answered, "I'm sad because I'm going to die."

How do we explain these things? Even though she is in the last stages of Alzheimer's, she emerges from her confusion. She *knows* her life is slipping away. Today she feels tired, weak. Is the end nearing? I don't know. But with Kenna's help, she is learning to navigate across that mysterious bridge between life and death, body and spirit.

Knowing Before *We* Know ...

"Your mother said something unusual," Hawa tells me as we eat dinner together. "When she woke up from her nap this afternoon, she said, 'I can't stop him. He won't listen to me.'"

Hawa continued, "Your mother was so clear I decided to ask her who, and she answered, 'My brother.' Then she sank back into her crazy chatter again."

Hawa pauses, her fork halfway to her mouth, "I never knew she *had* a brother."

"Oh, yes," I answer, "Swante. He was the third-born—the only son. He stayed on in Minnesota."

We finish dinner and decide which Monday night shows we want to watch and give Mom's strangely coherent conversation no more thought.

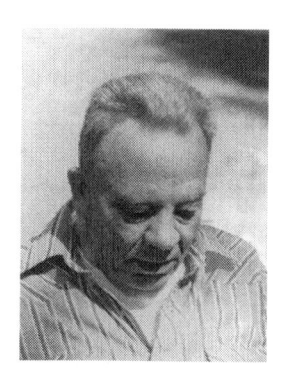

I'm upstairs trying to work in my office-closet when the phone rings. I pick it up on the second ring. "Barbara?" I hear an unfamiliar voice on the line.

"Yes?" I answer, mentally scrolling through my brain's voice-recognition data bank.

"This is Pat," the voice goes on. *Oh! Now I'm connected—it's that flat Minnesota accent.*

"Well, hi there," I answer, surprised by the unexpected call. Being distant cousins, we only exchange annual Christmas cards. I've never received a phone call.

"Swante died."

I hold the receiver motionless, my whole body falling into a strange silence.

"When?" I ask.

"Yesterday afternoon."

~ ~ ~

I hang up the phone, stunned. *Swante was passing over,* I realize, when Mom told Hawa, *"I can't stop him. He won't listen to me."* She *knows* she has lost her only brother.

I feel like I've stumbled into an Alice-in-Wonderland world—one that cannot be replicated by scientific experiment or by wiring Mom's brain to neurotransmitter monitors.

She not only became lucid, she relayed information I wouldn't receive for another 24 hours. How is this possible?

This event, more than any other, convinces me that Kenna's work is real, that psychic communication is possible, and that the world is much larger than what our limited senses sometimes perceive.

Now I walk into Mom's room. "Hawa," I say, still in shock. "Mom's brother died on *Monday* afternoon."

"That's when your mother told me," Hawa gazes over at her, sleeping peacefully. "Well," Hawa adds with a laugh, "she's better than AT&T."

It's My Turn

[After having Mom in my home for over a year, things fall apart. Hawa, who has become part of our family, suddenly leaves for Sierra Leone. Her mother has had a stroke. I go through caregiver after caregiver. They don't show up; they have sick children or broken-down cars; they need to be trained; I find myself caring full-time for the caregiver. Exhausted, I finally face my own reality. Grieving deeply, I move Mom into a small near-by group home. I feel bereft. My home feels empty. But I realize I truly need a break...]

~ ~ ~

"Sandra," I call my sister. "Mom's doing pretty good at Reddick's, but I want to take an RV trip. It's been so long since I've been away."

"Hey, that's great. Come out here!"

"That's the point. It'd take two months to get out there, see a few national parks, and get back. I don't feel comfortable leaving Mom for that long."

I don't mention something else. I feel like I'm being hit with an intuitive brick: *Get Elsie to Sandra. Mom needs to say good-bye to her.*

"Look, Barbara, it's my turn. You've done all the caregiving, but I'm the firstborn. I feel guilty you got stuck with all of this. You should be able to travel if you want. What if we move Mom out here to a group home?"

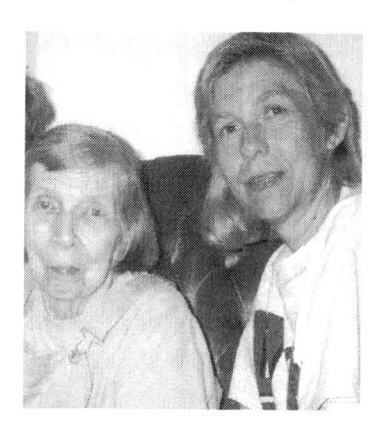

"Sandra," I admit, "taking care of Mom isn't the easiest thing—even to see her. She's pretty much bedridden. It can be depressing. She's wasting away." I find conflicting emotions inside me about Sandra stepping in as caregiver. *What if Mom dies and I am not there?*

After all these years, I feel like I have lived with a baby monitor that keeps beeping at me—*my mother's needs, my mother's life*. I can't separate myself from it.

When I started her care management, I never realized that caregiving permeates your whole life.

Do I believe anyone can take as good care of Mom as I have?—and had *I taken that good of care?* I give myself no gold medals. I haven't forgotten all the missed calls: the disastrous testing, the neglect in the shiny gleaming Alzheimer's facility, the delay in getting emergency care after the broken hip. *Do any of us ever take good enough care of our loved ones?*

"Barbara," Sandra insists. "it's my turn. Let me research this and see if there's a place near me."

"Hey, Sandra, before you do that, let's get Kenna involved. It'd be an interesting experiment. Maybe Mom can help us make the decision. I mean, she can stay right here at Reddick's if she's okay with me not being here for 2 or 3 months. Let's ask *her* and see what happens."

"Okay," Sandra, equally curious, agrees.

How About Seattle?

"Kenna, I'm worn out," I admit. "I just want to get away for 2 to 3 months.

"I've talked to Sandra about this. I was trying to come up with some options. Sandra decided she'd like to step in if we could get Mom to the West Coast. She'd put her in a group home near her."

"Well, *that* would be a big step for your mother," Kenna noncommittally answers.

"You know," I add, "I would never tell Sandra this, but I keep having this feeling that Mom *needs* to be with her—to make sure Sandra's okay before she leaves.

"Anyway," I continue, "we've come up with three choices. We want you to ask Mom which she prefers.

"She can stay at Reddick's, but she won't see me for 2 or 3 months. Or she can move to Seattle to be near Sandra. Or (this the surprise choice) she can move back to her Florida home and Hawa will take care of her."

"I thought Hawa was in nursing school now that her mother has passed away," Kenna interrupts.

"No, she's taking a break to earn more money."

"Ohh!" Kenna exclaims. "That's the choice *I* would make. Florida and all that sunshine."

I don't tell Kenna I'm absolutely certain Mom will *not* pick that option. She'll want to be near one of her daughters.

~ ~ ~

Elsie: *Hi, Kenna. I know who you are. I feel you.*

Kenna: Well, Elsie, Barbara is going to be away for 2 to 3 months and she is making plans for you. She has some ideas and wants you to decide.

So here are your options: You can stay where you are, but you won't be seeing Barbara for a long time. You can go to a group home in Seattle to be near Sandra. Or you can go back to your own home in Florida and Hawa will take care of you.

Elsie: *I don't like that. My daughters wouldn't be there. I don't want to move.*

Kenna: But if you stay here, you will be alone for 2 months.

Elsie: *I don't like that.*

Kenna: You don't want to be alone?

Elsie: No. I like having people around. It's more exciting than living alone.

Kenna: Well, here are two other options. Seattle near Sandra ...

Elsie: Or ... ?

Kenna: You can go to Florida and stay with Hawa and Sandra and Barbara will visit when they can. You would be alone with Hawa. She would take good care of you.

Elsie: I like Hawa.

Kenna: She likes you. It was her idea to take care of you in Florida.

Elsie: I like Florida.

Kenna: When Barbara gets back, you could live near her again, but it might be in a new place [not the Reddick's Group Home].

Elsie: Why can't Barbara see me now?

Kenna: She's traveling.

Elsie: Oh.

Kenna: Barbara needs to travel and do some new things.

Elsie: Barbara's always doing new things, isn't she?

Kenna: Yes, I guess she is. She works hard to take care of you.

Elsie: I know. I'm thankful.

Kenna: Well, Elsie, what's it going to be?

Elsie: I don't want to be away from my daughters.

Kenna: I understand. Do you think you want to go to Seattle?

Elsie: Seattle sounds like it's near the sea. Have I been there before? I like to be practical. I also want to be thrifty. How practical is this? Barbara is the planner. What does she think?

Kenna: I don't know. Barbara wants you to decide.

Elsie: And Sandra would visit and play music? I like to dance. I miss dancing. I dance in my dreams around and around. I could dance all night but I get tired.

Kenna: I don't know, but Sandra would visit.

Elsie: Well, let's go. [Kenna "sees" her kicking up her legs in excitement.]

Kenna: Are you sure? You could be with Hawa.

Elsie: She's not my daughter.

Kenna: I know. Sandra's children could visit you too sometimes.

Elsie: I'd like that. When would we go?

Kenna: If you move, it will be by August.

Elsie: Absolutely meaningless to me.

Kenna: Well, soon. I'll tell Barbara what you said and I guess you'll go to Seattle unless you change your mind.

Elsie: I'd like my family to be near me. I'm old, aren't I? How old am I?

Kenna: Well, you're in your eighties.

Elsie: Do you have to go?

Kenna: Yes, but I'll be back.

~ ~ ~

Does Mom truly participate in the decision to move to Seattle? Frankly, I don't know.

She doesn't remember Seattle, and Sandra doesn't play the piano or sing. But she adamantly refuses the Florida option.

She knows Hawa is not her daughter. She tags me correctly as *always doing new things* and being *the planner.*

As I believed, she clearly states *I do not want to be away from my daughters,* later adding, *I'd like my family near me.*

And then there's the trademark Elsie: *I like to dance ... I dance in my dreams.*

Ever ready for adventure, she kicks up her legs and uses the phrase I've heard her say so often, *Let's go!*

But in no way does Mom express an end-of-life *need* to be with Sandra.

My strong intuitive sense might be pure imagination. But of course, we didn't ask her *that* question and won't know the answer until a psychic asks her, years later, when she is on the other side. ...

Takeoff Time!

Kenna: Do you know what's going to be happening, Elsie?

Elsie: Of course I know. Does Barbara think I am an old fuddy-duddy?

Kenna: So you understand?

Elsie: Yes, I'm going to see Sandra.

Kenna: Yes, you're *flying* to see Sandra.

Elsie: Ahhh, I always loved to fly, didn't I? Well, I'm ready!

Kenna: Okay, you leave in about a week.

Elsie: Are you coming?

Kenna: No, but I will visit you there like I do now.

Elsie: People will be coming to say good-bye, won't they?

Kenna: Yes.

Elsie: I don't like good-byes.

Kenna: Well, just in case they don't see you again.

Elsie: I understand.

I'm Just Fine!

[Hawa and I fly Elsie first-class nonstop from Maryland to Seattle. Sandra and her husband Ed meet Elsie, complete with balloons. They have their van ready with a mattress, pillows, and blankets. Too excited to sleep, Elsie shines for the next day, then crashes and sleeps for two.]

~ ~ ~

Kenna: So how was it, Elsie?

Elsie: I had FUN! [She is laughing.] *It was like the good ole days, but I was the Commander-in-Chief.*

Kenna: Are you okay at the new place?

Elsie: Well, I don't get very hungry. I have no reason to die as long as I am having fun. I have no fear. I really feel good. I have always kept my heart to myself, haven't I? Anyway, now I am content and I hope my children are as well.

Elsie: I have been busy thinking about Barbara and Sandra. How is Hawa? I hope she had a good time.

Kenna: Is there anything you want to tell them?

Elsie: YES! Get me out of here! No, I am just joking. Just let them know I am fine.

~ ~ ~

Not only is Mom safe, she's absolutely giddy about her new adventure.

I, on the other hand, feel a sense of loss. My role of caregiver ended, it takes me time to not automatically run daily mental care lists through my brain.

My routine disrupted, a certain emptiness creeps into my life.

I turn my attention to planning my RV trip—which will include a visit to see Mom in about six weeks.

I've Lived My Life the Way I Wanted

Kenna: So how are you, Elsie?

Elsie: I'm feeling fine. I'm happy. I know Barbara was worried but everything is fine. I'm so happy to see so many of my family. In the end, they are all you have left, you know.

There's more activity here so I'm not so bored. I'm something of a spectator although it's not so much seeing as sensing and knowing. It's a different way and quite useful.

Actually it can be cunning and fun. People can't be sure what I see or don't see. Only I know. In a way, I like that! Like being a spy without an eye. Of course, I've got no one to give information to. That's the other part of the joke, you see.

Kenna: Do you have any messages for Barbara?

Elsie: I know Barbara wants to know about Sandra. Well, we're all fine. I know Barbara will be back.

Kenna: She's traveling and coming to see you soon.

Elsie: Good. We'll dance. I've always liked the change of scenery. New place, new people. Of course, I miss people but I'm not so attached as many are. Live and let live, I always say.

Kenna: How did you get like this? [get Alzheimer's]

Elsie: When I broke my hip, I got very depressed and didn't want to be alive. My brain was getting weaker and weaker which was depressing too. Yet the brain reaches a point where depression becomes an unknown. [Kenna interprets this to mean you don't realize you are depressed.]

Kenna: Well, that is your *mental* level.

Elsie: This is where I'm a goner!

Kenna: Elsie, what do you want?

Elsie: I think I want to think straight and stay focused.

Kenna: [sensed a fear in Elsie that if she didn't have Alzheimer's, she would be very depressed and that was the more unbearable option.]

Kenna: What's in your heart, Elsie?

Elsie: I'm content. I like it here. It's good to have family. I lived my life the way I wanted.

~ ~ ~

Kenna's conversation with Elsie reassures us that moving her close to Sandra was a good decision.

The shake-up animated Mom during those initial weeks once she recovered from travel fatigue. *I've always liked the change of scenery. New place, new people.* Certainly a trademark Elsie comment. Her satisfaction with life (*I lived my life the way I wanted*) brought back memories of "Elsie-isms" written in her journal:

> I have seen what I want to see
> I have done what I want to do
> I am just riding out the rest of my life.

> I'm going to be
> all I can be
> as long as I be.

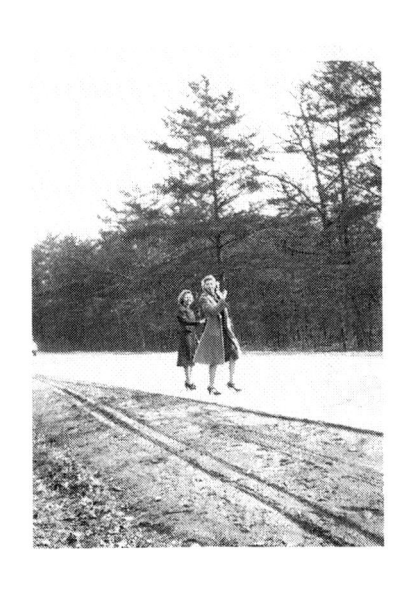

41

But then Elsie unexpectedly explains, *I'm something of a spectator. It can be cunning and fun ... like being a spy without an eye.*

As her daughters, Sandra and I well knew how much she used invisibility to watch over us.

Once, Sandra *thought* she was "borrowing" our school lunch money.

She seduced me into a great treasure hunt. When I burst into the kitchen, enthralled with my riches—Sandra with bulging pockets behind me—Mom, in a flat Finn voice from behind closed doors, mutters, "Put the lunch money back, Sandra." Sigh. Instead of a horse whisperer, we had a mother whisperer.

At the first Maryland group home, she stationed herself unobtrusively in a tiny portico aside the living room where she could see and hear, but not be seen.

She was right: *People can't be sure what I see or don't see.* But as she now tells Kenna, *without an eye* (a working mind), she has *no one to give information to.* And that is the *other part of the joke.*

As I listen to Kenna describe Mom's depression, I recall that moment in rehab after her hip surgery and my certainty she was *not* ready to die. Yet she tells Kenna that she *did* want to die.

But which Elsie was it—the depressed woman who was losing control over her world, or the essence-of-Elsie whose spirit still seemed strong and so unready to die?

In the end, Mom offers Kenna an intriguing insight: *The brain reaches a point where depression becomes an unknown.*

Having Your Own "Mental Travel Agent"

<u>Kenna</u>: Did you enjoy Barbara's visit?

<u>Elsie</u>: Yes, but I don't remember when she's coming back. I'd like to go on a trip like that.

<u>Kenna</u>: Like Barbara's?

<u>Elsie</u>: Yes. I love to travel.

<u>Kenna</u>: You can travel in your mind. Just say where you want to go.

<u>Elsie</u>: You're right. I can. All I need is to go to a Mental Travel Agent. [She laughs.]

<u>Kenna</u>: What's in your heart today?

<u>Elsie</u>: I like it when my grandchildren visit.

<u>Kenna</u>: What about when the angels visit?

<u>Elsie</u>: Yes, but I like to see my family more.

<u>Kenna</u>: Angels are family too. You have your own family of angels.

<u>Elsie</u>: I never thought about it like that.

<u>Kenna</u>: It's true. You have your own angels and I have mine. Of course, some angels visit everybody. So you can have your angels visit any time. Just call on them.

~ ~ ~

While in earlier sessions with Elsie, Kenna mentions angels in passing, now she begins to be very focused on connecting Mom to her angels. She helps her to see them.

My sense is that Kenna knows the end is nearing and wants Mom to have a safe and easy passage to the other world. Kenna is taking the lead here.

For the first time, she is not just listening to Mom but guiding and instructing her.

Why So Quiet, Elsie?

Kenna: So what are you thinking about?

Elsie: I'm thinking I like it here. Where's Barbara?

Kenna: On a trip. In Colorado.

Elsie: Will she be coming back soon?

Kenna: I'm not sure. I think so. Do you want to say anything to her?

Elsie: I miss her.

Kenna: Is your family visiting more often?

Elsie: Yes, and they brought fruit.

Kenna: But Elsie, you don't eat fruit.

Elsie: No, but my mind does.

Kenna: Elsie, you seem quiet. [This is the most quiet Kenna has ever seen her. She's not talkative.]

Elsie: I've settled down here. I'm ready for another adventure.

Kenna: You can go on adventures in your mind. Look to your left, Elsie. See the angel?

Elsie: Yes.

Kenna: She can take you wherever you want to go.

Elsie: Angels are light and fluffy. I like much more substance!

~ ~ ~

Later, as Kenna shares this conversation with me, she asks, "Does your mother tend to be indirect? She's not acting like herself."

It's a strange question but I try to answer it. "Oh, Mom was the master of indirectness," I admit, thinking back to her child-whisperer skills.

"But really, I think it's a generational thing. You know, women of that era grew up in an unequal world. How were they supposed to get their way? Sometimes she drove Sandra and me crazy."

"How did she do that?" Kenna asked curiously.

"Well, one time she worried about Dad's health.. Sandra and I were both married, but she called us to give us our part in a 'script' she had put together." I started laughing.

"It was kind of ... 'Okay, Sandra you say this, then Barbara, you stop by the house later in the week and say this'—and Mom gave us our speeches.

"It sounded absolutely insane to me. 'Why don't you just tell him what you want?' I asked. But I already knew the answer—they never had direct conversations about Dad's health."

"Did it work?"

"I think so—I honestly don't remember. But he *did* go to the doctor a few times in his later years. So maybe...."

"Well, I keep sensing your mother wanted to tell me about something bothering her. She was just too quiet. That's where I got this feeling of indirectness."

"I guess we'll just have to wait and see," I tell Kenna, a bit worried.

Dancing with the Angels

[When Kenna connects the next time, she continues to be concerned that Elsie is so unnaturally quiet and not talkative the last time. It is the worst she has seen her.]

Elsie: *I'm not feeling well.*

Kenna: How so?

Elsie: *I've been thinking about the meaning of my life. Was I a good mother? Did I make the right decisions?*

[Kenna senses something has happened at the group home that has depressed Elsie.]

Kenna: I'm here to cheer you up. Depression is an option you don't need. What is going on? What happened?

Elsie: *I don't know.*

[Kenna continues the energy-healing work on Elsie.]

Elsie: *I feel better already.*

Kenna: Let's remove all this heaviness from your heart.

Elsie: *I'd like to dance now.*

Kenna: Have you been talking to the angels?

Elsie: *No.*

Kenna: Why not?

Elsie: *Oh, I don't know what to say.*

Kenna: Just talk to them like you talk to me. They're here to be your friends and to help you. Just tell them what you would like.

Elsie: *Okay.*

Kenna: Think of the angels as a delegation from another country.

[Kenna finishes her energy work by filling Elsie with Light.]

Elsie: It feels like sunshine.

~ ~ ~

"Kenna," I ask, "what happens when you are filling Mom with Light? What does that mean?"

"Well," Kenna pauses, searching for words to explain something that can't be seen, "we're all connected to an eternal Source. Even in the Bible, it says, 'Let there be Light.'

"We have ways of expressing it, like saying, she lit up the room.

"The Light within us can be expanded until it kind of overflows. When I allow that, it starts pouring out of me in all directions. It's like I'm being filled with Divine Essence and then I channel it into your mother so she too can experience it."

"Like sunshine," I answer, remembering my own experiences with Kenna. I feel as though my whole body is *saturated* with Light, as though it cannot hold one more molecule of it.

But Kenna's effort to focus Mom on angels fails to work. Mom sidesteps, saying *Oh, I don't know what to say*.

From my perspective, this is vintage Elsie—she isn't interested. I am left wondering why Kenna talks with Mom so much about angels. Is she preparing Elsie to go? Does she see the end nearing? She doesn't tell me.

After listening to Kenna, I call Sandra who tells me, "Remember the woman in the other bedroom?"

I vaguely recall a bedridden woman so small and frail as to be barely noticeable. "She died a couple weeks ago."

I call Kenna back. "I wonder if Mom got depressed because, in some way, she sensed that death and knew that her time was coming?"

Neither of us has an answer.

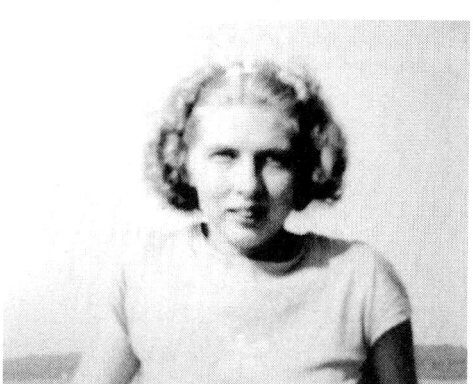

I See Clearly Now

[Kenna sees Elsie's heart beating very slowly. But that is just the way it is at that moment. The guides tell her the issue is not her physical health, but a kind of nervous agitation—the death of the other woman has triggered a lot of issues for her.]

Kenna: What's going on, Elsie?

Elsie: *I don't know.*

Elsie: *You know my brain got clearer and I began to see myself more clearly.*

[Kenna senses that she sees her true situation.]

Elsie: Tell Barbara I love her. I'm sorry I didn't show it much.

Kenna: So what do you want now, Elsie?

Elsie: Oh, I'm tired now. I just want to rest. Tell my family not to worry. I'm okay.

~ ~ ~

"Barbara," Kenna tries to explain what's happening, "all her life, your mother has been unable to let her real thoughts out. This is the way her body reacts to the fact that the woman's death has upset her."

"I don't understand."

"If we don't release our emotions, then our body holds onto them and releases them some other way—like an illness.

"Your mother had the opportunity to talk to me last Sunday but she didn't take it. That's not her way. It's not her personality. So she had to release it some other way. In a way, she is calling attention to herself.

"I get a strong sense," Kenna added, "that she needs more attention when something like this happens."

"So, that death really affected her," I reply wondering how it can be avoided in a home for the elderly.

"This is definitely a reaction to what has happened there." Kenna explains. "It is on her mind, and heavy in her heart."

I realize once again—I just cannot make death go away.

The Emergency Room

"Your mother is having difficulty breathing. She seems to be in pain," Stacy, the group home owner, alerts Sandra.

"I'll be there in 10 minutes," Sandra hangs up the phone, grabs her keys, and yells to a coworker. "Something's wrong with my mother. Tell the boss," and she flies out the door.

Stacy greets her at the door. "I've called 911."

Sandra walks into Mom's room. She's struggling to breathe, her skin is pallid. She looks frightened. Sandra grabs her wrist, feeling for the pulse. It's shallow and rapid. Sandra begins to croon to her while they wait. "Mom," she leans over whispering, "they're on the way. You need to go to the hospital."

Elsie looks lost and confused. She grips Sandra's hand.

Watching her struggle to breathe totally unnerves Sandra. She can hear the siren coming down the road, growing louder as it turns onto the gravel driveway. She hears the door opening, the sound of heavy feet walking rapidly to the room.

The paramedics move her aside and start taking vitals. Their voices seem so loud. "Is there a 'Do-Not-Resuscitate' order?" the lead medic raises his voice. Sandra jumps.

Stacy says "Yes," and races out of the room.

"Let's get her into the ambulance." the medic orders. Minutes later the siren is screaming down the driveway. Sandra calls Ed. "Mom's having an emergency. I *need* you!"

"Stay put. I'll be there in 15 minutes. I don't want

you driving."

Sandra calls me. "Barbara, Mom's having trouble breathing. The ambulance has just taken her to the hospital. Ed's picking me up. It looks bad."

Emotions start colliding inside me. I am 3,000 miles away from Mom. I can't take charge; I can't take care of her. All I can do is ask questions. "What happened?"

"Stacy thinks it may be pneumonia. I'll call when I know something."

We hang up. It is 7 p.m.

What is going to happen? I walk around the living room. I sit down and try to pray. I can't. I go to the phone. *I need to get there.*

Then I realize there *is* one way I *can* be with Mom....

"Kenna," I talk rapidly into the receiver. "Mom's been taken to the emergency room. Sandra says she's having trouble breathing. Can you connect with her?

"Okay, Barbara. I'll check to see what's going on."

I Want to Rest

Kenna: I'm here, Elsie.

Kenna: Are things going to be okay, Elsie?

Elsie: I don't know. [She seems scared and confused.]

Kenna: Well, let's try to hold on for Barbara to get here. You're giving them a good scare."

Elsie: Yeah, well I'm good for something.

Kenna: Who is with you now?

Elsie: Just the usual crew.

Kenna: Barbara is coming.

Elsie: I'd like to see her.

[Kenna sees that she can go either way. It seems that

Elsie has vomited.

Whatever is wrong, Kenna sees that she will have a recurrence. At this moment, Elsie does not know what she is going to do.]

~ ~ ~

"The doctor needs to talk to you, Barbara. You have the medical power of attorney."

"Give me an update, Sandra," I hear my voice sounding strangely tinny and high.

"She's not going to make it," Sandra answers in a choppy, heavy voice as unnatural as mine. "Here's Dr. Fisher."

"Is this Barbara Erakko?" I hear Dr. Fisher identify himself over the phone.

"Yes," I answer tensely, gripping the receiver.

"You have medical power of attorney, is that correct?"

"Yes."

"Her lungs are about 70 percent filled with fluid. She's too weak to cough. She's in septic shock."

"What does that mean?"

"It means all her organs are shutting down. She's experiencing severe abdominal pain. We can do heroic measures to keep her alive or palliative care to make her comfortable.

"What do you want us to do?"

"Can you keep her alive until I get there? I'm getting the next flight out."

"Then we'd have to start heroic measures."

I silently hold the receiver thinking of Mom. *I always promised you no pain—oh happy death.* The silence drags on.

"Are you there?" Dr. Fisher asks. "What do you want us to do?"

I start to cry.

"I swore I'd do everything in my power to protect her from pain—that's what I've tried to do for her all these years." I had a hard time going on.

He waited. I could feel anger rising up in me—anger at *death*. I'd never see her alive again. I'd never get there in time.

"Oh happy death," I say in a defeated quiet voice. "No heroic measures."

"Okay, Ms. Erakko. I promise you, we'll make her comfortable."

No Wonder People Die

<u>Kenna</u>: What do you want, Elsie?

<u>*Elsie*</u>: *I sure am not going to hang around in a lot of pain. I will tell you that! I won't put up with this nonsense. All this coming and going. I want to rest. No wonder people die. To get some rest!*

[Kenna clears the energy between Mom, Sandra, and me. Whatever happens will be okay. Angels are with her.

Kenna tells her what to do and how. When all of that is set, Kenna gives her benediction.]

~ ~ ~

Kenna calls me as soon as she disconnects from Elsie. "Sandra needs to stay as calm as possible. Your mother is scared and confused.

She adds, "It's not her intention to die. She may recover but it could happen again. Tell Sandra if she thinks your mother is dying, tell her to go to the Light. She is confused and she needs to stay focused."

I burst out crying. "The doctor called me. They can't save her without heroic measures. I can't get there in time. Kenna," I feel a sorrow so deep I cannot find the bottom of it, "I'm going to lose her. I can't even say good-bye."

"You can talk to her, Barbara. Tell her what's in your heart. "

"I know." *But really I don't. I'm not a psychic. I'm a daughter.*

~ ~ ~

Elsie is now slipping away so fast there's not even time to admit her to a hospital room. The emergency-room staff rolls her to a quiet, curtained area. Sandra and Ed are with her.

I call Sandra. "Kenna says for you to tell Mom to head toward the Light."

"Okay," Sandra promises.

Saying Good-Bye

"We're going to start an intravenous morphine drip to make her comfortable," Dr. Fisher explains to Sandra. "She's in septic shock and in abdominal pain."

Sandra now knows too. Mom will die.

~ ~ ~

I'm trying to pack and getting nowhere. I stand in the middle of the bedroom and say to my daughter Lisa, "I can't think." I feel myself going hysterical.

Lisa starts pulling clothes out of my closet. Never have I been so glad to have my daughter staying with me. She's taking charge. She finds airline numbers, and locates a 10 a.m. nonstop flight to Seattle.

I sit numbly in my mother's Queen Anne chair. Hours are passing. I cannot sleep. I pace in nervous agitation. Lisa keeps vigil with me. I turn to her. "I'm starving! I need to eat."

"Double-T Diner is open," she tells me.

"But it's after midnight."

"They're open all night. I'll drive."

As I hand her my car keys and we walk out the door, I mentally connect with my mother. I tell her matter-of-factly: *Let me know if you're passing over.* I don't say it with any adamancy. Not in a demanding way but in a bereft way. I am heartbroken, my mother is dying, and I will not be with her. I never imagined such a thing. Always, always, I felt that I would be by her side to see her off. As Lisa whips the car down darkened roads past neon signs of closed businesses, all I can think is this: I am 3,000 miles and an airplane flight away.

~ ~ ~

Lisa and I arrive at the all-night diner. I am surprised at how *busy* a diner can be at 2 o'clock in the morning. I see lots of young couples, kids sleeping on vinyl booth benches while parents socialize at Formica-topped tables with old-fashioned juke boxes perched on them.

We sit down at our table and open our laminated menus when someone taps me on the shoulder. I look up. I see two college-aged couples. They are laughing. One of them asks if I will sing for them. Just at that moment, I notice there's no restaurant table for them. Instead, three chairs have been placed, two backed against one. "What?" I ask, perplexed.

Lisa pipes in. "Mom, they want to play musical chairs."

"Oh," I hear myself saying. It makes absolutely *no* sense to me, but nothing makes sense. My mother is dying. I can't get to her. I'm sitting in a restaurant at some god-awful hour. The place is hopping alive and I can't figure that out either. Why *not* sing?

"Okay," I answer, and launch into my version of "Coming 'Round the Mountain." That eliminates one guy.

I move into "I've Been Working on the Railroad." A girl goes down. Now only one chair remains. "I'll have to close my eyes," I tell the remaining boy and girl. "If I watch, I'll make sure the girl wins."

I shut my eyes and begin to sing one of Mom's favorite songs, "You are My Sunshine." As I sing, I feel all the sadness falling from me. *This is the strangest thing,* I think as I continue to sing. *I'm so happy. I almost feel like I'm flying,* and am overcome with ecstasy.

I yell "STOP," and look to see who won. The boy sits triumphantly on the chair, doubled over with laughter.

I turn back to Lisa. "What time is it?" I ask.

She glances at the restaurant clock. "It's 2:30 in the morning, Mom." All my anxiety is gone, completely gone. I don't know what to make of it. All I had wanted, with every particle of my being, was to be in Seattle. Now I feel my body letting go of trying.

When we return home, I feel peaceful, quiet.

I go to my jewelry box to get Mom's bracelet—the one with the enamel pins identifying all the delegations she had been in charge of while a Protocol Officer. I have worn it to every major family event once Mom could no longer attend—weddings, graduations, birthdays. Now, a funeral.

The next morning, at 7 a.m. the phone rings. *Did Mom make it through the night?* I wonder, assuming she has because I've gotten no calls from my sister.

"Barbara, Mom died last night at 11:30 p.m."

"What?" I say in disbelief. I sink into a chair. "Why didn't you call me?"

"It wouldn't change anything. I knew you'd need your sleep before traveling today."

I hold the phone in my hand, my sister on the other side. The silence goes on and on as I feel my mind go absolutely blank, my body numb. Finally I shake myself and say, "Sandra, I've got to go. I've got to get to the airport. I've got to leave." And I hang up.

Lisa comes to my side. "Mom died at 11:30 last night," I tell her.

She stares at me quizzically as though thinking about something. "Mom, that's when you were singing for those kids in the restaurant."

I stare at her uncomprehending. Then I realize ... 2:30 a.m. in Maryland would be 11:30 p.m. in Seattle.

57

I return in my mind to the moment I began singing "You are My Sunshine"—how ecstasy filled me, how I felt so happy, as though *joy* rushed through my body. *She was passing over,* I thought to myself, absolutely awestruck.

I have been told that when people talk to us from the spirit-side, they identify themselves so that we'll know who they are. Mom *loved* music and dancing. It was in her bones.

I had asked her to tell me if she passed over. She used *music* as the way I would know ... absolutely.

She didn't need her chair anymore.

[The next day]
I Feel Great!

Elsie: *Kenna, I DID IT! You were right. A lot of people met me and I have been busy. But I have come off by myself to talk to you. I feel great! Everything works! My brain! My legs!*

Of course, it is not that I have them [she has a body of light], *but you know what I mean.*

I <u>told</u> you I was ready for another adventure. Tell Barbara and Sandra I am happy. I wasn't expecting things to go like this. All so quick. But I am happy and I feel great. [Under her breath,] *I should have done this sooner.*

It all worked out fine. I got extra time with Sandra. Tell Barbara not to worry. I really didn't die alone.

Kenna, you have been with me as Barbara's representative, and all the angels were there. It was a big send-off. And now I can <u>really</u> fly!

But I am just spending time with old friends right now. BYE! ... And she disappears.

It's All Right Now
[four days later]

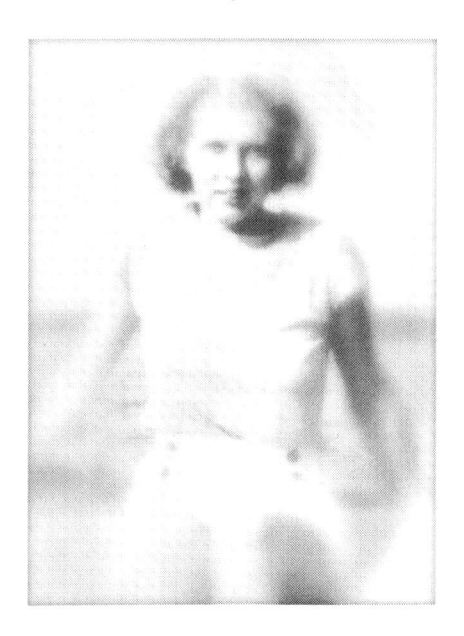

Kenna: How are you?

Elsie: I'm just fine. I'm still having a good time but things have calmed down a bit—like after a cocktail party.

Kenna: Well Barbara wants you to know that she's at peace and she's delighted you had a good crossing. She says to say hi to these people for her. She would like to visit too.

Elsie: Oh, she will. Her time will come. Tell her I want her to be happy. We loved her. We always did. We just lacked understanding, didn't we? It's all right now. Barbara understands. Tell Barbara I am nearby and I will see her Saturday. Can you imagine that all that is left are those ashes? [Kenna sees a twinkle in her eye] *I got the better deal, didn't I?!*

~ ~ ~

What makes this reading particularly interesting is that I have not told Kenna we plan to hold the memorial service on Saturday, nor have I mentioned that Mom was cremated.

There was no reason to tell her.

Mom has become the messenger.

Pushing the Pocket

By 2008, eight years had passed since my mother died. My grieving felt muted—like the final notes of a long symphony that slowly faded into silence. During the 13 years of Mom's struggle with Alzheimer's, I mourned the slow loss of the woman I knew as mother. But intertwined with loss, I felt awe.

Mom seemed to experience a very special portal between two worlds. She remained earthbound by this debilitating disease, yet she seemed to be crossing over to spirit.

Over the course of years, her body and spirit—so interwoven in life—seemed to slowly unwind until the two strands separated completely. Mom became all spirit, not needing her body any more—and then she died. Quickly.

I wanted to ask her questions ... because there were so many unanswered ones.

One day, I simply asked myself, *why not*? Why not interview Elsie now on the other side? Why not have reputable psychics connect with her? I viewed it as a scientific experiment. I would choose five, based on recommendations from people I respected. I would experience a reading with each one myself. Then, if satisfied, I'd ask them to connect with Elsie and ask her two questions:

1) What was her experience of Alzheimer's, from the inside out, and

2) What would she want caregivers to know?

By the end of the year, I had done four interviews with Elsie, all conducted by women. Of course, I asked Kenna to be one of the participants.

"Why?" Kenna questioned.

"Because nobody could really see inside her head while she was going through the disease," I explained. "We have no idea what it *felt* like to be experiencing it." I rush on. "Since you were connecting with her while she was alive, and you connected with her right after she died, I see no reason why we can't interview her for the book I want to write."

I met the next psychic when I moved to Poulsbo, Washington. We became friends. One day Angelita asked my help in moving some items with my van, and I agreed. As a thank you, she offered me a free psychic reading.

Now I had never had one. I considered Kenna's work with my mother and me to be energy healing. Never had I allowed anyone to *read* me—and I felt nervous. But unable to think of a polite way to refuse, I found myself sitting in her room.

My experience from that day and others taught me that our souls, or higher spirits, have a purity of intent that often get ruffled by day-to-day ego-based concerns. We truly are unable to see the forest for the trees. A good psychic sees past those disturbances, allowing the inner self to express its true desires and path. Usually the sign of a good reading is that the recipient feels heard, listened to in a very deep and profound way.

So my second candidate for interviewing Elsie was Angelita Rae.

Eventually I moved to Hannibal, Missouri. A small river town known mostly as Mark Twain's childhood home, I became close friends with a woman renown for supporting historic home preservation, and the arts. Eventually I learned she had worked with Kay Wagner, a psychic in New Mexico, for decades. She often shared what transpired in a reading.

I made contact with Kay.

I slowly learned that each psychic has a unique way of receiving information. Kay explained, "I don't connect as though I'm having a conversation. I see visual images and get impressions.

"It feels like instantaneous thought and it comes in clumps rather than verbatim conversations. It literally *leaps* through me. I don't have time to think about it, let alone judge or edit it.

"I also get emotional information. I *feel* it in my body. I will laugh or giggle or be filled with sadness. I also see gestures, like the wave of a hand."

Kay became the third person to interview Mom.

The fourth and last woman lived in Florida.

A close friend of my ex-husband Bill, Donna Edwards not only conducted readings, she also taught others how to increase their telepathic abilities via seminars and Internet conferences. As with the others, I was curious as to how she received information.

"Well," she explained, "I connect with several levels of guides.

"When connected with very highly evolved spirit guides, I feel stronger energy coming through my body as though I'm being pulled into a higher vibration.

"Once I'm connected, information just comes through. If I sense the answer is too general, I will stop and wait—sometimes I will then receive very specific information."

Now I had experienced four interviews but two years would pass before I would find the fifth person...

~ ~ ~

For my last interview, I wanted a man. I wondered how a man, whose entire life perception is obviously quite different from a woman, would receive Elsie—and how she would express herself.

Unfortunately, my network yielded nothing and eventually I forgot.

In 2010, my ex-husband Bill showed me a website he had designed for a London-based medium, Ronald Hearn. Immediately I felt an inner *click* and emailed him. He agreed to be my fifth interviewer.

My connection to Ronald was unusually "clean" in the sense that we had absolutely no contact. All he received from me were the emailed questions I wanted him to ask.

With the other psychics, I could at least talk on the phone or be with them in person, making it possible that I'd interject information—even though my intent was to be as scientifically neutral as possible. In the end, every psychic—including Ronald—established their own credibility.

They refused payment.

It would make little sense for them to waste personal time to give me a fake psychic reading. And an Internet search would yield nothing more than a gravesite photo.

With all the psychics, Mom used certain identifying characteristics. In all instances, she came through *strongly*, which I am told is somewhat uncommon. And she often spoke in a pithy way, quite like in real life.

She invariably mentioned how she loved dancing and the piano.

Lastly, the information cross-correlated very well between the psychics, making it credible that one person, Elsie, was indeed connecting to us.

I also learned subtle differences exist between psychics and mediums—not in their innate ability but in the way they refine it.

A psychic, generally speaking, sees their role as message transmitter. Often the person coming for a reading has concerns about *this* life so the psychic focuses on that.

A medium on the other hand *specializes* in connecting you with loved ones on the other side. They hone their ability to pick up concrete details about that person's *life* so the person receiving the message can decide if a connection has indeed been made.

With decades of experience, and international recognition, Ronald Hearn wrote several books about his experience as a medium. Not unsurprisingly, Ronald Hearn provides extraordinary proof of a connection to Elsie.

He doesn't literally *see* persons who have passed on or hear them speaking, but receives impressions.

"I find myself able to describe people and situations which I could not normally know about," he explains in one of his books. "I would never expect to get a hundred percent success. In many ways, [this work] is like looking for gold dust, and before the prospector can find a few grains of gold, he must first wash away all the dirt and unnecessary things from his pan."

Ronald's information was the last piece of the puzzle. His information is interwoven into the summary that follows.

So, had a cohesive picture emerged?

Of course the proof lies not in the technique but in the information. In culling through the five transcripts, I found five basic categories of information coming through:

- Her personality: in various ways, Mom says or shows herself in distinct ways unique to her.
- Dying Process: in four separate accounts, she gives remarkably similar descriptions.
- Alzheimer's Experience: all accounts have a strongly similar emotional feel but each psychic receives different metaphors to describe the experience.
- Advise for Caregivers: all accounts have strong similarity.
- Alzheimer's from a Medical Perspective: remarkably, while I never once asked the psychics to question Mom about this, she interjected her comments about it in several places.

1. Personality

As mentioned earlier, the psychics I used tended to concentrate on the *messages* that Mom gave and only coincidently gave concrete details about her persona.

For example, Angelita notes, "Your mother tends to be very intelligent. She's very analytical at times—that's how she dealt with her emotions. If she could *understand* them she wouldn't get carried away too much."

Later Angelita adds, "She liked to dance. It was the one time she didn't have to be on guard. It was the closest thing to flying—letting her defenses down, being free and spontaneous."

Unknown to Angelita, Mom told Kenna almost precisely the same thing when still alive: "Dancing is not just exercise for the body; it is a way to clear the mind too."

Kay provides identifying information of an emotional nature. When asked about the testing for Alzheimer's, Mom didn't mince words. "I was totally disgusted with it."

Kenna provided numerous pieces of information in the year she worked with Mom—her love of music and the piano, the fact that she loved flying while Dad preferred boats, and so on.

Ronald, on the other hand, emphasizes identifying characteristics. Like Angelita, he sees that, "Your Mom is quite an intelligent lady." He goes on: "She was always ready for things."

I immediately remember seeing Mom jumping out of her seat, saying, "Let's *go!*"

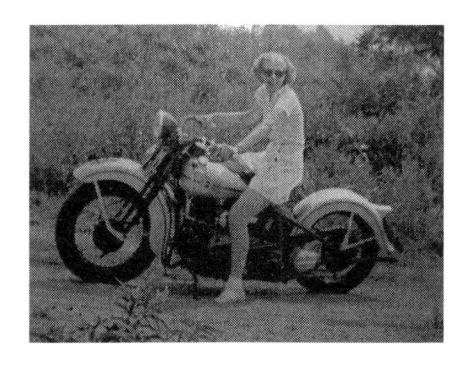

He continues giving descriptive information. "She has sparkling eyes. I think she could look at people and through people somewhat.

"She was not a person to feel sorry for herself. She would make the most of it and get *on* with it."

I remember when Dad died. She resolutely buried his ashes at sea within days of his death, and got rid of everything—his clothing, his tools, his ham equipment—except his battered leather wallet, which we found hidden among her belongings.

Ronald, recording his sensations of her onto the CD he sent me, sometimes presents his information as questions. "Did she play the piano? She seems to come through with what I call lovely piano music. Happy memories of piano playing."

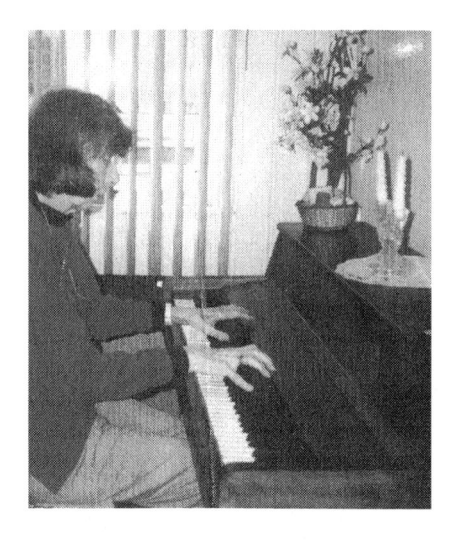

Then he offers the single most startling identification of any of the five psychics: "She says Herbert is here watching on—her husband, of course."

This takes me by complete surprise. *Could he have learned this some other way?*

But then, I look at the facts: He's in his eighties. He's done this work for decades. He's written three books on the subject. He's had hundreds of clients—and he's doing this reading for *free*.

He turns to Mom's feet. "Before she passed over, she had difficulty with her feet and shoes—some difficulty with getting the right shoes."

Mom, suffering from bunions and hammertoes, bought so many shoes Dad nicknamed her Imelda Elsie after the Philippine First Lady Imelda Marcos who owned nearly a thousand pairs.

Ronald also tells me, "She is giving me a strong message about flowers—something funny she did with them."

Sandra reminds me of the petal-less bouquet Mom handed Lady Bird Johnson.

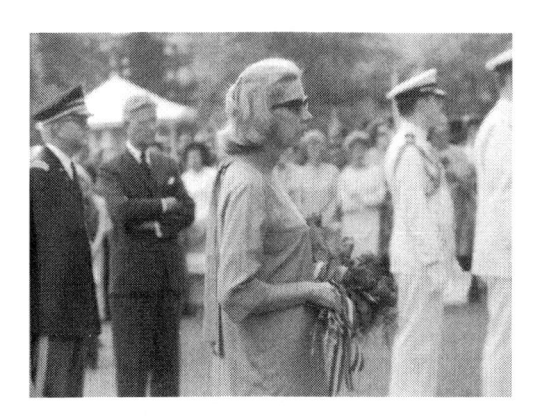

I delight in these concrete details but am clueless when he sees something funny about umbrellas. Then I recall he explained that spirits do not operate in *our* time. A message may refer to the past, present ... or *future*!

Lastly, he notes that, "She tends to wave her hands around a lot when she is speaking."

I don't remember that until—months later—I read an entry in *my own journal* about her flapping hands!

I feel Mom has worked hard to identify herself so as to establish her credentials. She adds one more extremely important detail—how she died.

2. Dying

I wasn't by Mom's side when she died. I only know that from calling 911 to death took about four hours.

And of course, she had *no* way of communicating with the family even though Sandra and Ed were beside her. Yet to four psychics, she describes the experience almost exactly the same way.

First, we have Kenna who connected with her hours after her death. Mom exclaims, *I wasn't expecting things to go like this—all so quick! But I am happy and I feel great.* [Under her breath,] *I should have done this sooner.*

While I hadn't specifically asked psychics to query Mom about her dying, she naturally discusses it as part of her experience of the disease.

When Angelita talks with Elsie about it, she says, "Your mother just lit up saying, *I was ready to go!*" Angelita gets this a-ha feeling from Elsie of completion— and that the moment she got that, she knew she was ready. Very easy.

Kay picks up the acute abdominal pain Elsie experienced. *Boy,* Elsie says, *that was REALLY painful.* Then she shows Kay how the death occurred: *Whoosh! Similar to a bird. Quick. Pop! Without aggravation.*

Ronald simply explains, "Your mother was happy to be released.

"She said it was a wonderful experience to wake up and find oneself in another dimension, another world, but without pain, without problem, with only clear thinking, and to meet up with loved ones."

When asked to interview Mom on the other side, Kenna returns to this topic and Mom tells her:

> *Finally the time is right, the opportunity is there, the door flies open, and you know you'd better run fast to catch that train!*

3. Alzheimer's Experience

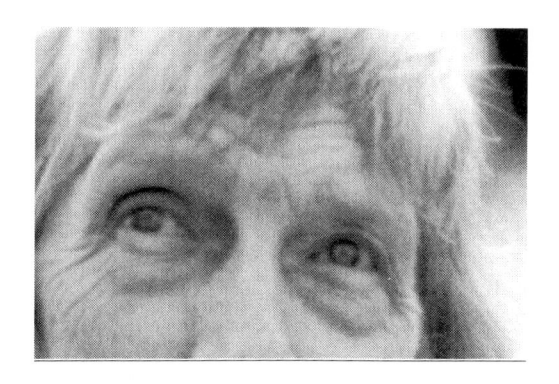

If, having reached this point, we are convinced we are actually talking to Elsie—and I am—then what she has to say about Alzheimer's and caregiving takes on significance. We can peek behind a locked door—for who can communicate with a living person whose mind has literally been wiped clean?

In virtually every instance, Mom vividly describes her fear, frustration, and anger as she entered the downhill slide into Alzheimer's.

She tells Angelita, *It scared the hell out of me.* To Donna, she admits, *It was frightening*; to Kay, *very frustrating, aggravating, and frightening.*

To Ronald, she explains, *It is like a feeling of wanting to escape from an unhappy situation. Sometimes people with Alzheimer's get very angry and unhappy—as though one is trying to get out of prison. Anything to get away from this disease!*

I well remember Mom's anger that ranged from frustration to all-out fury.

These might be defined as the beginning stages of the disease, when she could observe her own diminishment with frustration, anxiety, and fear. None of what she says here surprises me. I also observed these stages.

She shows several examples of how it felt to her.

Angelita sees Mom in a room filled with objects looking for something she can't remember but will know when she gets to it. Mom explains she won't know *how* she knows, but by going through each of those little pieces, she'll get to what she really wants.

It's like when you know that you know a word or a person's name but you can't retrieve it at the moment you want it. Then you reach the point where you can no longer search because you no longer remember that you once knew the word. It's like someone hands me a piece of paper, but my mind can't grasp what it is and what to do with it.

It's not exactly memory; it's discernment. It was as though I had thoughts floating in my head and I couldn't understand which thoughts were mine and which might be coming from some place else.

I clearly remember the day I brought in a photo of Mom to show Hawa. She exclaimed, "Oh Elsie, you were really *HOT!*" and held it close to Mom's eyes but the link was broken—the image, the paper, the memory itself all severed from Mom's memory.

The beginning stages of Alzheimer's are filled with trauma both to the one experiencing it and the caregiver. Fear, frustration, anxiety, and loss overwhelm everyone.

At this stage, anyone would unanimously agree—it is the most wretched, awful, unbearable disease imaginable.

I remember *wanting* Mom to "progress" to the next stage of the disease where caregiving would be easier. But once she arrives there, I no longer have any way to communicate with her. A door between us closes.

But now, that locked door opens...

It was like entering a fog, she explains to Kenna.

To Donna she says it was like *stepping into a void and I didn't know if I would fall deeply into it*. She uses different phrases: *A bit of darkness, lack of clarity, unfamiliar territory, not being able to see clearly or navigate through it.*

This reminds me of a time when I was working quietly in the basement and my husband, thinking no one downstairs, turned off the light.

Certain that I could navigate using my memory, I didn't say anything. I walked to where I thought the stairs would be and immediately began crashing into objects.

Soon I was completely disoriented. Without a single point of reference, my world suddenly became meaningless, my memory useless. Unlike Mom, I could yell for help. She could not.

Kenna sees two big panes of glass—almost like patio doors that slide over one another when open so they look like one door, but these have a distance between them and will never touch.

Angelita also sees sliding glass doors—Elsie on one side and knocking but the people inside don't see her.

Eventually Mom leaves the anger and frustration behind. Why? Because emotions need a cause, and cause needs memory.

Without memory, the link between cause and emotion dissappears. She also leaves the caregivers, Hawa and me, behind. We can continue to care for her physically, but the emotional link is broken. Now she begins to cross over.

At first, I was puzzled. Mom's eyes would focus on the wall or ceiling, gesturing and talking. When I asked, "Who are you talking to?" she always gave me the name of a deceased friend, family member, or co-worker.

I clearly remember the day Mom pointed across the room, stating, "There's Eddie." By this time, I agreeably waved, saying, "Hi, Eddie" to the empty air. Eddie had been Dad's best friend. Then Mom pointed to the space next to him. "There's Wayne."

Now *that* stopped me in my tracks.

Sandra and I never told Mom that Eddie's son, Wayne, had died of a stroke at the age of forty. Yet Mom pointed to the only two members in that family who had died—she didn't acknowledge any of the family still alive.

I was having conversations with people, with loved ones, Elsie now explains to Donna, *and I could communicate better on that level. I lost touch with communication on the earth plane, but on the other side, all could be understood without the use of vocal cords. There was a language, so language was used, but so much understood at a high level, it felt as though language was not necessary.*

From Mom's perspective, she saw herself drifting from the shore of her remembered life.

In many ways, she explains, *there was a gentleness about it,* she says, *as though I was being eased out of one world and into another without fear.*

It was a world of peace, serenity, escape from the thought process, escape from a human reality one does not want to face. It became more and more welcome to retreat into another plane of reality, she explains to Donna.

I reached a point where it was almost like flipping a switch. One moment I would be in human reality, and then the switch would go off and I'd be in the other reality. It was like having one foot in one plane—and the other in quite a different place.

Over time, she preferred the other reality: *I saw glimpses of Light that were beautiful. I felt I was being lifted into a higher place with much gentler energy than human consciousness. I saw glimpses of people I had known before. It was as though the real world was becoming muted.*

My escape from the real world became more and more pleasurable. The more I wasn't present in my human body, the more I experienced living heaven on earth.

Eventually it got to the point that being forced back into human consciousness jolted her.

She tells Donna, *I felt more comfortable in the other reality. Those around me, in their well-intentioned attempts to bring me back to the present—that was intrusive.*

I had landed in the other reality very safely and that became more familiar to me. I felt a bit less safe when jarred out of that—perhaps by someone speaking to me or taking care of my needs.

She tells Kay precisely the same things.

I was communicating with the other side and was further and further into the other dimension. It was quite natural. The rest didn't matter—just the quality of energy around me. [Loud] *voices,* [harsh] *touch—just as some sounds turn you off—it could make me cringe.*

Elsie takes a different tack with Ronald. She spends more time explaining how it *feels* to be in a blocked, crippled mind.

"Your Mom wants to make it clear that the soul or the spirit, the life force, is a thing of clear thinking. There is no deterioration. "

She says to Ronald, *The soul* knows *it cannot get out of the physical body. It is blocked off. Therefore it tends to cross over. Of course it does not cross over completely, but it is trying to escape from something it knows it cannot fight, it cannot cure. So there is a natural pulling over.*

Later she repeats herself, *The soul is* fine, *but it is being blocked off.*

The idea of "lights out" doesn't really portray the true reality of the disease. On some level, the soul sees and observes—but can no longer speak through the diseased mind.

In my understanding, when the mind is healthy, the soul uses it as a conduit for self expression and all is well. But as the mind slowly diseases, the soul's energy becomes trapped, imprisoned—yet the *urge* to be connected remains strong, healthy, and utterly unchanged.

This blockage forces the soul's energy to find another outlet for expression. Although the spiritual side was always accessible when her mind was healthy, Mom had little interest in connecting to it—life itself was much more exciting and interesting. Only when trapped does she finally quiet down and allow the always present spiritual energies to interface with her soul-self.

Angelita explains the blockage using a different image. In her healthy life, Elsie made choices: "It's like she's in this bubble and as long as she's there, no one else's energy can penetrate—and none of her energy goes out.

"Your mother worked hard to control her world. Alzheimer's 'scared the hell' out of her. It's like the first half of her life was about living one way; the second, about healing from that.

She needed to be in control and be rational. So what does she experience? Irrational. No control. No mental level to deal with that.

She ends up learning how to be with things on a spiritual level."

As Elsie herself said to Kenna, *The Alzheimer's experience is an inter-reality experience—being in a place between two realities—this world and the "other world." It is actually a l-o-n-g journey between the two worlds. We know where we have been, and we're in no hurry to get where we are going!*

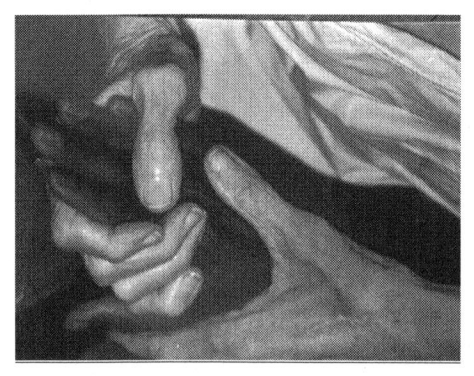

4. Caregiving

In the beginning stages of Alzheimer's, much advice exists for the caregiver. The first recurring frustration between caregiver and the afflicted concerns forgetfulness. "I just told you that." "Don't you remember, we can't take the escalator." "You just ate!"

In ordinary circumstances, in *healthy* circumstances, the one being addressed would re-direct, recall, and somehow the situation would resolve itself.

Not so with Alzheimer's. The afflicted one has no *way* of recalling, and often angrily, with toddler-like determination, insists that he or she is right.

Eventually caregivers learn tricks. They stop saying, "I just told you," because it never works. They redirect. "Well, we'll take the escalator in a couple of minutes. I need to look for a sweater." "Oh, you're hungry. How about a snack?" What works for the two-year-old now works as well with the beginning stages of Alzheimer's.

Once the dementia really sets in, the caregiver loses all the cues and clues. That brings on a completely different set of worries, guilt, and anxieties.

Here Elsie offers a great deal of compassionate advice, based on her own experience. She affirms, for the first time, the value of Kenna's telepathic presence.

I was very happy to communicate with Kenna, she tells Donna. *Kenna was a bridge between the two realities because she was on earth but she could communicate with me.*

She calmed me down, and let me know everything was okay. It really helped me to accept where I was instead of struggling. It gave me tremendous peace. It became exciting to be able to communicate at a higher level what I was feeling.

When Kenna reconnected with her eight years later, Elsie comments, *That is why someone like you is so nice because the Alzheimer's patient has gone into an interior world and "interior communicators" are needed. Life goes on in this "other world." It's sort of like we're all in the same house but in different rooms.*

She adds later on, *It was a relief to know I had someone to talk to, someone who could really communicate with me. It's nobody's fault—Alzheimer's patients or caregivers—it's a new language that needs to be learned because really, it's like two people from different countries.*

79

She expressed gratitude for Kenna similarly to Kay: *Kenna—her way of being present—was helpful in freeing me.*

But Elsie still remained tethered to the physical world. *People carrying this illness,* she explains, *become more sensitized to what is happening around them vibrationally. They sense who feels they are a burden.*

To Donna, Elsie goes into detail concerning why it is so valuable for caregivers to keep talking to those with Alzheimer's—even in advanced stages.

It is *not to elicit a response,* Elsie explains, *but to allow the caregivers to express what they are feeling towards the person. It may be an apology—I am sorry if you are picking up on my feeling burdened but I have a lot of stress right now. I'm having a hard time coping with losing you.*

Elsie suggests caregivers s*peak from the heart because people often don't do that. Families that have never touched each other's hearts find that there is so much anger and resentment left unsaid.*

She continues, *This is a good opportunity to fully communicate from their heart, their emotions, frustrations, disappointments. Allow* everything *to be communicated and released while the person is still on earth, and then when the person has parted, there are no regrets. Everything is said when the afflicted one is in a semiconscious state where it will not be hurtful but fully understood.*

I remember sitting by Mom weeping as I told her I could no longer care for her in my home. What she says affirms what I believed—that in a soul-to-soul way, we were connected.

When I asked Kay if I had been right in thinking Mom needed to see Sandra one last time before she could pass over, Mom said yes.

Kay saw her patting her heart as though her heart were opening several times, saying it was a *quick resolve*. Sandra admits she grew fonder of Mom even though lingering issues remained.

I also had my own experience when I told Mom that she would be moving out of my home. I talked to her as though she comprehended everything—and I was miserable with grief, and yet also relieved.

It seems that once Elsie began to live more in the spirit world, she could see the human condition more clearly, with more compassion. She adds that caregivers should not feel guilty arout seeking other care, be it a nursing home or hiring help.

In the advanced stages, she explains, *the person cannot distinguish family from people anyway. You reach a place of peace. You just want to be on the other side anyway and are not in a place of judgment or even awareness of who is giving you the care.*

But she does emphasize to Kay *one* aspect of caregiving that remains powerful even in advanced stages—touch and sound. *Touch is important,* she explains, *and the tonal vibration of the voice.*

She also comments that *Kenna's way of being present was helpful in freeing her to go when she was ready.*

Kenna did, in fact, prepare the way. She told Mom telepathically how to navigate in this quasi-spiritual realm. As Kenna connected with Elsie each month, she observed changes.

Very near the end, she saw Mom reach a moment of clarity—after another resident died—about the true reality of her condition. Before, Mom always enjoyed Kenna's visits. Now, Kenna saw her quiet and reflective. Later she told me, "It seemed as though your mother had made a decision."

Now Mom acknowledges Kenna *was helpful in freeing me to go."* All the preparation, showing Elsie her angels, clearing worries and concerns about this life, prepared Mom to depart. It was an unusual form of caregiving, but important, nevertheless.

With Ronald, Mom becomes quite specific.:

Caregivers have got to act or react to the people in their care with love and caring. They are called carers and that is what they must be doing.

It is very, very important—the attitude with most nurses, carers, doctors, all sorts of people—is that when people develop Alzheimer's, it is deterioration—but they don't think about the soul, the spirit, the life force within. They treat the physical.

Elsie asks Kenna, *Who is helping who in the end? One person is offering another an opportunity to serve, to become a true human* be-*ing while helping someone who is no longer* do-*ing anything. That is hard work.*

She continues, *The Alzheimer's patient is teaching so much in this stillness, actually even inviting the caregiver into it. It is no secret that that is where you find God—in the stillness.*

But she reserves the most reassuring message for Ronald.

Love, she explains, *is the* greatest *thing. It has to be the sort of love that will understand people's conditions, people's situations.*

She continues, *Barbara has a lot of love in her. She is very loving and caring. The more love you have, the stronger you will be—and if you do things with absolute love you cannot fail.*

She tells Kay, *Barbara's understanding and her freedom allowed me to be. There is such a pull from some family members to stay—such grief—it makes it more difficult for a person to just freely go.*

She also seems to imply that love is an important ingredient in addressing this disease. *Things can happen and go ahead, but with love, they can* really *go ahead, and that can* really *have a breakthrough. You know, love conquers everything.*

Personally I don't see how love could have healed or minimized Mom's Alzheimer's. I just felt I bought her time. My intuitive sense kept telling me, *she's not ready yet*—so my caregiver job was to support an extension of her life until *she* decided it was time to leave. Otherwise it would have been abrupt, like a premature birth into the other world.

What I wanted was a *natural* birth into the next world. So in that sense, I suppose, love *was* an important factor. It *did* allow things to go forward.

5. Alzheimer's as a Disease

Here, Elsie takes us across yet another portal. Personally, I didn't ask—or expect—Mom to talk about this, which means *she* is going "off-script." I had my agenda, but apparently she had one too, and they didn't entirely mesh. More specifically, I only thought to ask questions that I already had some opinions about—how she experienced Alzheimer's and her caregiving recommendations.

Consider the humor in this. Stubborn daughter that I am, I stay completely fixated on *my* questions. It never occurs to me that *Mom* might have some other topics she'd like to discuss. I never ask, "Is there anything else you'd like to add?" So I go through psychic one, psychic two, psychic three, psychic four—and still she can't crowbar her way into these tightly scripted, Barbara-directed interviews.

After two years of waiting, one last opportunity arises ... Ronald Hearn. And what does she do?

"I was watching television trying to relax," he later tells me, "and suddenly, it was like the TV was turned off. I could feel someone bringing through a whole lot of things about the other world."

Mom comes in with such force that Ronald has to stop what he's doing and write down her messages, even though his scheduled time to connect with her isn't until the next day.

Of course, I know nothing of this for the next several days, as Ronald burns a CD with the information from his reading and mails it to Hannibal from his London residence.

Every day, I check the mail anxiously awaiting its delivery, until one day the reinforced padded envelope arrives. I immediately tear it open, put the CD into my player and press PLAY.

Right away, he describes the strange events in front of his TV. Then, he diverts and takes time to describe Elsie, so I can be sure it is my mother giving the information that follows. I delight in all the detail he gives, laughing at some images and being awed by others.

At last he goes back to the message, and it begins with her words, *Alzheimer's is <u>NOT</u> a disease.*

I slam my thumb on the pause button, stunned, and mutter irately and loudly so Mom would be sure to hear me, *Then what the HELL is it?*

I feel my whole book whooshing down the toilet bowl of wrong ideas. A major premise of my writing has been that we should consider telepathic communication with loved ones suffering from any mental impairment.

But what if the information seems insane, crazy, and unbelievable? How could Alzheimer's NOT be a disease?

Feeling a bit tremulous, I push the PLAY button and continue listening.

To my amazement, she repeats this exact, precise declaration, not one or two times—but SEVEN times. So it's important, I reluctantly decide, to try to understand her point of view.

For the next several months I turn her message over in my head, replaying the CD several times. The other messages fit nicely with the psychic information I've already received, but this one remains enigmatic until I *really* listen.

Ronald relays Elsie's words: *The soul or spirit is normal and remains normal. It is the deterioration of the body and things that affect the blood. Things are out of balance, but the soul or life force is strong. It doesn't get older in the same sense as the body. It is the deterioration of the body in old age creating an imbalance.*

So that is Elsie's first salvo.

A couple of clues emerge.

First, the brain *is* bathed in blood. If that blood is no longer as healthy, as nourishing to the brain—if it has *imbalances* in it—certainly, it seems, the brain *will* suffer. Imagine the brain bathed in blood nurtured every day by fast food, sugary snacks, alcohol, lack of water, no exercise?

The human brain, though only two percent of the body mass, receives 15–20 percent of the blood supply.

Secondly, she continues to see the soul as utterly healthy. This appears to be very important to her—the *essence* of Elsie cannot be destroyed by this disease.

She continues, *Things are bound to deteriorate with age. Life has to run its course. But there are so many wrong diets.*

She gives Ronald the sense telepathically that diet, vitamins—that sort of thing—make a difference. In particular, Ronald relays, "I keep getting the feeling of *green*. A lot of greens connected with it. She doesn't seem to be saying people should eat a lot of greens, but that something taken from greens will be very important."

Ironically, shortly thereafter, I stumble across an article in the June 2012 issue of *Mind, Mood & Memory,* published by Massachusetts General Hospital, entitled "Green Tea May Help Conserve Cognition, Cup by Cup." *Well,* I decide, *it's green.*

In one of the innumerable studies now going on about Alzheimer's, this one finds that polyphenols, called catechins, in green tea are a potent antioxidant. It helps retard brain aging. Using words like "in some research," "suggests," and "may" to add cautionary notes, it reports reduced risk, slowed progression, reversed age-related loss, and repaired neuronal injury associated with aging.

More recently, in March 2015, a study by the Federation of American for Experimental Biology reports on the efficacy of green vegetables:

> "The researchers tracked the diets and cognitive abilities of more than 950 older adults for an average of five years and saw a significant decrease in the rate of cognitive decline for study participants who consumed greater amounts of green leafy vegetables. People who ate one to two servings per day had the cognitive ability of a person 11 years younger than those who consumed none."

Mom explains to Ronald, *The whole physical body has to carry you through life and it needs to be strong. But it deteriorates and that deterioration causes untold problems. Therefore, Alzheimer's is not a disease—it is an aging process that has to be dealt with and the only way is by building up the system.*

It seems as though she is giving the word *disease* a make-over. But the medical establishment, itself, has done a similar turn-around with regard to cancer, heart disease, diabetes, and obesity. In every case, evidence mounts concerning how strongly diet, exercise, and lifestyle affect these *disease* statistics unlike the AIDS *virus,* for example, which seems more intractable.

This is not to discount genetics or Mom's earlier comments that things are bound to deteriorate. It just suggests we can do certain things to slow, or possibly eliminate, the *causes* of it. But currently, virtually all medical thinking seeks a cure for Alzheimer's in much the same way pharmaceutical solutions are sought in the war on cancer.

Elsie comments, *They are not really working on the right thing in the right way. But they will get there. Alzheimer's is not a disease. It is something quite normal in its way in so far as aging goes—the big question is how to slow the aging process.*

If Elsie had made insights about the disease only to Ronald, it might have been easy to dismiss. But she also commented—without being asked—on the disease question with both Angelita and Donna.

She shows Angelita her resistance to putting a medical label on it and then tells her, *The jury is still out on whether this disease is even hereditary.*

To Donna she explains, *Alzheimer's is a disease of the times. It is physically caused by the erosion of the brain—both with over-chattering of the mind, and not taking care of the body.*

It is of these times, she adds, *because people are learning to live from the higher mind and to take care of their bodies. When that is accomplished, then people will be able to live heaven on earth without having to do it through the illness.*

I sometimes think how frustrating it must have been for Mom, on the spirit-side, to get the attention of her stubborn, truculent daughter.

I hadn't asked the *one* question she desperately wanted to answer. Even when she gives clues to Angelita and Donna, I ignore them.

Given one last chance, she blasts into Ronald's peaceful evening trumpeting, *Alzheimer's is NOT a disease*.

At last she gets my attention.

Conclusion

Alzheimer's invokes tremendous fear in all of us. We cannot imagine losing our mind because, as Descartes said, "I think, therefore I am." Mom reacted no differently than any one of us would, given this devastating diagnosis.

My mother entered this journey reluctantly and with anger. I entered, as caregiver, with trepidation as to what lay ahead. Neither of us expected anything other than a terrifying life-end experience.

Yet today, that story of dread seems so intertwined with transformation. I keep going back to the caterpillar. *If* I had consciousness as that furry, crawling, little being and I got a diagnosis that my body would soon be encased in a kind of woven plaque—*and* that my very body would *melt*—I would be filled with even more dread than a diagnosis of Alzheimer's.

But we, as humans, *know* the end of that caterpillar's story. One day the cocoon breaks open. The butterfly emerges, wings wet. It stands upon the broken tomb, waiting for air to dry its wings. Then it flies away.

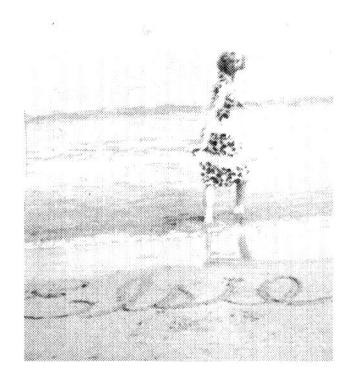

The story of Alzheimer's is not so very different.

When we are of sound mind, our soul or spirit-within uses all of our senses to express itself. We gesture; we talk; we use our eyes, hands, taste, and sound. Nothing blocks us from expressing the inner beauty that is ours.

But when Alzheimer's strikes, we find those portals slowly blocked, locked, walled off. Yet the soul within us has not changed. It remains healthy and vibrant ... but trapped.

Eventually it discovers an opening—an out-of-body place. Like a very long near death experience, it begins to cross over from the physical world to the spiritual world.

Mom loved her human life, perhaps more than most. She grabbed it with both hands. She absolutely did not want to leave. Alzheimer's, in a strange way, gave her all the time she needed to say her good-byes. It was a gentle and long bridge from body to spirit.

When she was ready, the door to Spirit wide open,

she simply flapped her soul-wings one time.

And was gone.

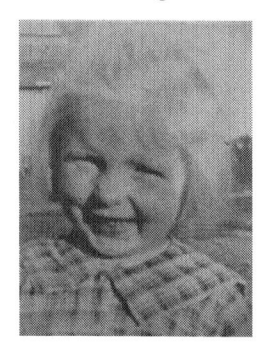

More to the Story...

You have now read excerpts from *Elsie at Ebb Tide: Emerging from the Undertow of Alzheimer's* focusing on the psychic aspects.

In the full-length book, Elsie, as U.S. Protocol Officer, hands flowers to first ladies Jacqueline Kennedy and Lady Bird Johnson, sometimes with disastrous results. She meets a queen and a pope, escorts an astronaut, faces an attempted assassination, and mistakes Nixon for hotel staff.

Meanwhile, Dad tells her, "You have the best damned job in the world; I'll take care of the kids." We are a blue-collar family with "an officer and a gentleman"—only the officer is my mother.

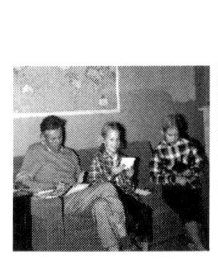

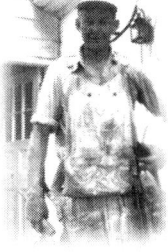

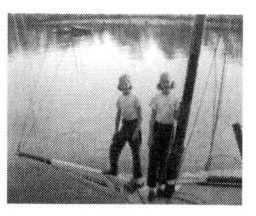

Growing up in the 50s with a father as our main caregiver certainly makes us an unusual family. Readers find themselves laughing, crying, and believing they have read a love story, a memoir, a book they don't want to end.

For me, it is a transformational story. It describes how I slowly but radically change my perspective on Alzheimer's.

I go from fear and dread to a sense of deepened love, awe, and even amazement. I come to see myself as a midwife, witnessing the rebirthing of my mother's soul into spirit.

As she loses her mind, she regains a child's sense of joy—I watch her eat pizza "for the first time" (in her memory-less world), and sing "When the Saints Go Marching In" as she marches into a doctor's office. I often like her world better than mine. I learn some things are not worth remembering: fear, anger, anxiety, guilt, sadness.

I finally come to believe that sometimes it is the relinquishment of our mind that allows us to regain the ever-present connection to our soul. Alzheimer's forces us to let go, and discover we are not lost at all—and never were.

The website, *www.ElsieAtEbbTide.com*, contains stories, photos, audio recordings, YouTube clips, and a full 25-minute program. Autographed and bulk-order discount copies of *Elsie at Ebb Tide*, this booklet, or the booklet, *Alzheimer's Transformed* can be ordered through the website.

The book, or booklets, can be used for Alzheimer's support groups, hospital ministry, hospice, or book clubs

Available at:

www.ElsieAtEbbTide.com

CreateSpace eStore

Amazon.com

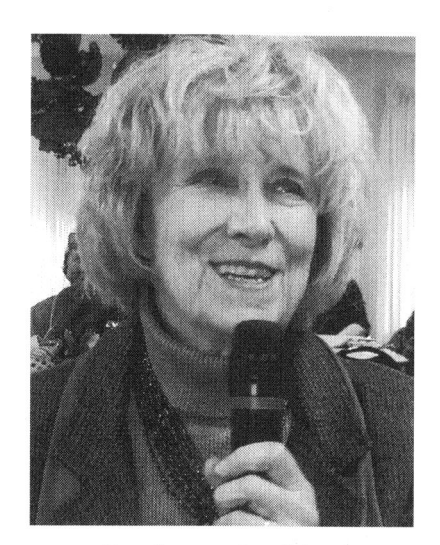

Barbara Erakko

comes from a technology-rich background, having designed information systems for the White House Executive Office as well as several Fortune 500 companies. While raising two daughters, she worked as a columnist for two newspapers, winning a national award.

Barbara is available for media interviews and speaking engagements. She also offers a full-hour program for local Alzheimer's support groups using her 25-minute DVD "Program of Hope," along with her booklet *Alzheimer's Transformed*, and a Skyped-In Q&A session.

For Booking Information,
Contact Lisa Pemberton
Pemberton Management Agency
(573) 795-2539

lisa@pembertonmanagementagency.com

psslisa@gmail.com

Elsie Julia Elizabeth Norlund Nurmi
Life Events

July 7, 1917	Born in Duluth, Minnesota to Jennie and Hjalmar Norlund
September 1923	Starts school, Finlayson, Minnesota, unable to speak English. She lives with her Finnish grandparents on their farm.
1927	Her father Hjalmar dies in a grainery accident. Her mother is pregnant with their fourth child, Alice.
May 31, 1935	Graduates with class of 17 as valedictorian.
September, 1935	Duluth. Becomes nanny and attends Duluth Business University.
March 1936	Duluth. Works for Great Northern Candy Co; acquires stenography.
September 1936	Oyster Bay, Long Island. Works as butler's girl for Howard Caswell Smith and attends NYC Business School.
September 1937	Wall Street. Works as Mr. Smith's substitute secretary.
October 1937	Lexington Manufacturing Co. Clerical. $5/week.

February 1938	North American Accident Insurance Co. $12/week.
October 1938	Kieckhefer Co., $16.25/week.
August 1939	U.S. Census Bureau. $26/week.
February 12, 1940	Marries Herbert Nurmi at Warrenton, Virginia courthouse.
August 1940	Social Security Board, Bureau of Old Age. Elmira, NY $25/week.
September 1941	Panama Canal, Washington, DC. $2,430/year.
October 1942	USDA Graduate School. Course in Government Contracts.
December 8, 1942	Takoma Park, Md. Buy home. $5,850.00
August 12, 1945	First Daughter, Sandra, born. Unemployed.
July 6, 1947	Second Daughter, Barbara, born. Unemployed.
September 1949	Atlantic Coast Line Railroad Co. $3,114/year.
December 1950	U.S. State Department. Office of the Chief of Protocol, Gifts and Decorations Office. Secretary. $3,275/year

1958 - 1966	U.S. State Department. Office of the Chief of Protocol, Protocol Assistant.
1966 – 1974	U.S. State Department. Office of the Chief of Protocol, Protocol Officer in charge of delegations to:
	Swaziland, Iceland, Paraguay, Mauritius, Tonga, Guatemala, Philippines, Berlin, Canada, Ecuador, England, France, Brussels, Netherlands, Germany, Italy, Spain, Portugal, Colombia, Brazil, Nicaragua (among others)
January 1975	Retired after 25 years at the U.S. State Department.
January 1980	Lake Worth, FL. Move permanently. Sell Takoma Park house.
April 15, 1987	Husband Herbert dies of complications from a stroke.
July 1992	Finland. Elsie, her sister Alice, and Barbara travel throughout country.
March 31, 1994	Finnish-American Rest Home. Elsie moves into assisted living.

February 1938	North American Accident Insurance Co. $12/week.
October 1938	Kieckhefer Co., $16.25/week.
August 1939	U.S. Census Bureau. $26/week.
February 12, 1940	Marries Herbert Nurmi at Warrenton, Virginia courthouse.
August 1940	Social Security Board, Bureau of Old Age. Elmira, NY $25/week.
September 1941	Panama Canal, Washington, DC. $2,430/year.
October 1942	USDA Graduate School. Course in Government Contracts.
December 8, 1942	Takoma Park, Md. Buy home. $5,850.00
August 12, 1945	First Daughter, Sandra, born. Unemployed.
July 6, 1947	Second Daughter, Barbara, born. Unemployed.
September 1949	Atlantic Coast Line Railroad Co. $3,114/year.
December 1950	U.S. State Department. Office of the Chief of Protocol, Gifts and Decorations Office. Secretary. $3,275/year

1958 - 1966	U.S. State Department. Office of the Chief of Protocol, Protocol Assistant.
1966 – 1974	U.S. State Department. Office of the Chief of Protocol, Protocol Officer in charge of delegations to: Swaziland, Iceland, Paraguay, Mauritius, Tonga, Guatemala, Philippines, Berlin, Canada, Ecuador, England, France, Brussels, Netherlands, Germany, Italy, Spain, Portugal, Colombia, Brazil, Nicaragua (among others)
January 1975	Retired after 25 years at the U.S. State Department.
January 1980	Lake Worth, FL. Move permanently. Sell Takoma Park house.
April 15, 1987	Husband Herbert dies of complications from a stroke.
July 1992	Finland. Elsie, her sister Alice, and Barbara travel throughout country.
March 31, 1994	Finnish-American Rest Home. Elsie moves into assisted living.

December 1, 1995	Alzheimer's Facility, Maryland. Elsie moves to Maryland assisted care.
August 9, 1996	Cooper Group Home. Elsie moves to three-3-bedroom assisted care unit.
October 1998	Barbara Taylor's Home. Elsie moves in with daughter.
November 1999	Barbara Riddick Group Home. Elsie moves to assisted care.
July 2000	Washington State. Elsie moves to assisted care near daughter Sandra.
October 13, 2000	Elsie dies.

Made in the USA
San Bernardino, CA
13 October 2015